Relieving Back and Neck Pain
What to do and why

Mark Smith B.Sc. (Eng), B.Sc. (Chiro), D.C.
Doctor of Chiropractic

Original Artwork
Ann Marie Foster B.A. (FA), M.A. (FA)
Artist

ISBN13: 978-1494897611
ISBN8: 149489761x

This book is not intended as a substitute for individual medical advice from a healthcare professional. The reader should not use information in this book to delay consulting a healthcare professional in matters relating to his/her health and particularly to any symptoms that may require diagnosis or medical treatment.

© copyright Mark Smith 2014
All rights reserved

Description

Mark Smith is a highly experienced chiropractor who has successfully treated many thousands of people with back and neck pain. Drawing on his many years in practice he has compiled the advice and exercises his patients have found most effective and easy to follow.

The book contains a wealth of useful information and practical strategies to help people suffering with back or neck pain. Much of the contents will also be relevant to those wanting to learn more about exercise and how to achieve good posture.

The book is arranged to ensure simple directions for relieving back and neck pain can be easily found. A more detailed explanation is also provided to give interested readers an understanding of the reasons behind each set of instructions.

Contents

Introduction   7

Chapter 1
Strategies for dealing with low back pain

What to avoid if you have low back pain   11

Acute low back pain
What to do when you start to experience back pain   13
Exercises for acute low back pain   14
Acute low back pain in detail   20
Managing acute low back pain   21
Use of medication   24
How long before you feel better   26

Chapter 2
Recurrent low back pain

What to do during a painful episode   27
What to do between episodes   27
Recurrent back pain in detail   28
Prevention   34
Exercises to increase low back strength
and flexibility can be detrimental   36
Exercises to increase low back stamina
and coordination are beneficial   39

Chapter 3
Exercises for recurrent or chronic low back pain

How to identify the best exercises   43
Exercises   45

Chapter 4
Sciatica (back related leg pain)

What causes sciatica	53
Treating sciatic leg pain	55
Exercises	56

Chapter 5
Relieving long-standing chronic back pain

Stage 1, Self help	65
Stage 2, Seeking help from a therapist	66
Stage 3, Further investigation	67
Stage 4, Pain management	69

Chapter 6
The common causes of back and neck pain

Anatomy of the spine	75
Back and neck pain - where does the pain come from?	76
Muscle injuries	77
Ligament and intervertebral disc pain	77
How facet joints cause back and neck pain	80
How sacroiliac joints cause back pain	81
Factors that slow recovery in ligament and disc injuries	82
Osteoarthritis	83
Can being overweight cause back pain?	83

Chapter 7
Making changes to work and other daily activities

Reducing sitting	85
How to adjust an office chair	86
Positioning laptops correctly	89
How to reduce the negative effects of sitting	90
Lying – finding the best position	92
Bending and lifting – what to avoid	94

Chapter 8
Pain in the middle and upper back

Restriction and lack of movement as causes of pain	97
Loosening exercises	98
Pain to one side of the spine and/or radiating around the rib cage	112
Pain between or around the shoulder blades	113

Chapter 9
Relieving neck pain

Avoid looking down	115
Acute neck pain	115
Should I exercise my neck?	118
Chronic long term neck pain	120
Headaches and dizziness	120
Exercises for reducing neck stiffness	121
Pain in the arm, hand, shoulder or between the shoulder blades caused by a neck injury	125

Chapter 10
Posture

The benefits of good posture	127
Adjusting posture in the hips	128
Improving the walking action	133
Correcting upper body alignment	136
Improving neck alignment	139
Relaxation – how it helps good posture	141
Breathing Exercises	141
Can stress cause back pain?	144

Chapter 11
Healthcare professionals - what they offer

Chiropractors, Physiotherapists and Osteopaths	145
Your Family Doctor	149
Orthopaedic/Spinal surgeons	152

Chapter 12
Additional exercises and information

Exercises for flexibility and good posture	157
Sit ups	177
Strenuous exercise, warming up and winding down	179
Using heat or cold to encourage healing	180
A few final words	182

Relieving Back and Neck Pain
What to do and why

Introduction

Most of the people I treat with back or neck pain would like to relieve their pain themselves. Many have tried various methods to alleviate their pain such as, advice from the internet, magazine articles, or approaches that friends have found useful. These self help efforts prove by and large unsuccessful because advice or received suggestions were not appropriate for their condition.

Frequently the strategies or exercises patients are using are totally inappropriate for their condition and without them realising they are making their complaint worse. Many of my patients with back or neck pain would not have needed treatment had they known the correct things to do themselves, at an early stage before their problem became chronic.

Understanding your injury and learning how to manage it is vital in assisting recovery.

In this book you will discover

How to use posture and strategies at work to help reduce pain in the back and neck.

How to help prevent further injuries once you have recovered.

An understanding of how injuries occur.

An exercise regime you can use yourself.

How to use the body more efficiently thereby increasing energy to enable you to enjoy a fuller life.

A wide range of self help approaches exist to help people with back or neck pain. However, many regimes particularly for chronic, long term problems, require professional assessment and supervision in order to be successful. Without professional help there is the risk of worsening your back or neck by following aggressive exercise programs. I have therefore focused on exercises and advice which in my experience most people can safely attempt without supervision. The exercises I have chosen can be integrated easily into your daily routine causing least disruption.

Many years spent in practice treating thousands of people, has provided a wealth of opportunity to identify the information and practical advice patients find most useful and easiest to follow. I therefore have my patients to thank for the choice of exercises and advice I have included in this book.

It would be unrealistic to claim that the advice in this book will alleviate every problem. Some people for instance will require more individual support from a professional. However, from my experience of treating patients with a wide variety of problems, the majority of people with back or neck pain will gain significantly from the advice given here.

How to use this book

Each section has concise and helpful advice which can be located easily by those with back or neck pain. In response to requests from patients for a fuller explanation I have included a detailed analysis. This may be of interest to those with long term problems.

How to select advice and exercises that suit you

The benefits of some of the advice and exercises may not be immediately obvious. My advice for those with chronic, long term problems is to read the book cover to cover, then select the advice and exercises that you can manage and feel comfortable with. Practising just a few of the recommendations in this book regularly will increase understanding and awareness of the body, and encourage you to try more of the exercises and advice, bringing long term benefit.

Chapter 1
Strategies for relieving low back pain

What to avoid if you have low back pain

In cases of low back pain unless there has been some impact on the body from a fall or car accident for instance, the bones are not normally damaged. In most types of back pain it is the muscles, ligaments or inter-vertebral discs where injury is most likely to be located. This injury normally involves some form of overloading of these structures causing some parts to become strained and damaged. When this happens the tissues become inflamed and sensitive. This is why after any injury it is important not to overwork the injured area of the body so inflammation can subside, and damaged tissues can start to heal and knit back together.

Stiffness and the guarding reflex

In most injuries the body will try and protect the injury by tensing up the muscles around the injury to immobilise it and prevent further stress on the injured tissue. This process is known as guarding. The effect of guarding combined with the effects of localised inflammation will cause the injured area to become stiff and feel less flexible. It is important to be aware that the feelings of stiffness you normally feel following an injury are a reaction to the injury and not the source of the pain. It is also important to let the body's natural healing mechanisms do their work, and avoid using the injured area too much or subjecting the injured tissue to strain.

Avoid activities that stretch or strain the injured joint

The best way to avoid over stressing the damaged tissue and assist the body's natural healing mechanisms, is to avoid activities that hold the injured joint in a stretched or strained position. This occurs when the joints are bent or twisted. I have listed those common activities (pg 12) which hold the joints of the low back in a strained position, bent forward or backward.

Common activities that strain the low back by causing the joints to be bent forward

Bending forward
Lifting
Sitting
Any exercise from the sitting position e.g. cycling, rowing, and any gym exercise done from the sitting position
Stretching forward
Stretching the ham strings/back of legs

Common activities that strain the low back by causing the joints to be bent backward

Bending backwards
Lying on the front
Sleeping on the front
Any exercise done lying on the front e.g. swimming on your front

If you have a back injury, limiting or avoiding these activities will reduce the workload on the damaged area and increase its ability to heal quickly.

Acute low back pain

What to do when you start to experience low back pain

Try not to worry. Most episodes of low back pain settle naturally.
The least aggravating activities for the low back pain are walking about and lying down.
When lying down, lie on your side (placing a pillow between your knees often helps) or lie on your back.

Avoid lying on your front. Lying on the front often aggravates low back pain.
If lying down is the most comfortable position, try to stand up and walk about for short periods as well, but avoid doing this too frequently because getting up and down every 5 minutes will jar your back.
If moving about eases the pain, remember to take rest periods lying down as well.

Avoid sitting. Most types of low back pain are aggravated by sitting.
If you have to sit, sit high up on a stool or a cushion so your hips are above your knees and your thighs slope downwards.
If you have to travel in a car try reclining the seat back, which often helps.

Avoid activities where you are standing still. Standing still usually aggravates low back pain.

Avoid activities that aggravate the pain such as bending or lifting.

If you can't find relief from pain in any position, making it difficult to sleep or relax, or if your symptoms are not improving within 2 or 3 days seek advice from a healthcare professional (see chapter 11).

Exercises for acute low back pain

Usually the safest exercises for people to do themselves are those that involve gentle movements of the joints, but avoid taking the joints into a stretched or strained position.

Walking – good for low back pain

For people with an acute injury, stretching and many other types of exercise may stress the damaged areas of tissue that are trying to knit together. If a damaged joint is overworked it can impede or interfere with the healing process. Walking is one of the safest exercises for people with back pain and widely recommended. Walking although gentle, puts enough loading on the body to help maintain fitness without excessively straining the joints in the back. The gentle, natural movements of walking eases tension in joints and stimulates the movement of fluids that help disperse inflammation and provide nutrition to the joint tissues.

Exercise

Basic pelvic exercise – good for low back pain

The point of this exercise is to cause a gentle repetitive motion in the joints in the low back, increasing movement and circulation.

To start lie on a comfortable surface with your knees bent up. Place your hands palm down at each side of your waist with the fingers slightly under the hollow of your low back. Without tensing or using too much effort, flatten the hollow of your back by moving your low back down towards the floor. Don't rush, take 2 or 3 seconds and relax, letting yourself follow the movement.

Towards the end of the movement you may feel tension across the front of the pelvis. If you feel this tension, do not go any further. If you don't feel this tension go as far as you can gently without straining.

At this point hold for 1 or 2 seconds then let your back relax up again.

You can do 10 or 12 repetitions any time during the day as long as you leave 1 or 2 hours between each set.

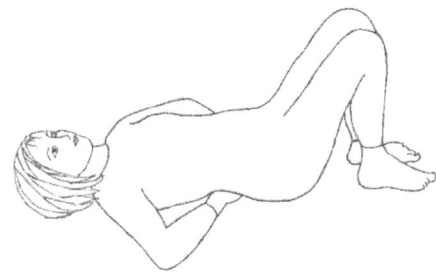

This exercise can also be done lying on the side if that is more comfortable. Lie on whichever side is more comfortable and place the uppermost hand behind your back.

Exercise

Knee rocking – good for low back pain

To start lie on your back on a comfortable surface with your knees bent up. Lift one knee at a time and hold them one in each hand with your arms straight and relaxed and the knees together.

In this position, if your back feels stretched or uncomfortable don't do this exercise until your back has improved enough so that you can hold this starting position without aggravating your symptoms.

If you can lie in this position comfortably then slowly rock your knees towards your face. Use your arms to do this, not your leg muscles, so your back remains relaxed. At some point your low back will start to pull tight and start to feel stretched.

As soon as you begin to feel the low back stretching stop, pause for 1 or 2 seconds, then relax back to the starting position.

Remember this exercise aims to gently move and mobilise your back to help gently loosen it and disperse inflammation. It is not a stretch. If your back is very acute and inflamed continued stretching may make it more inflamed. However, if you repeatedly move it without stretching you can loosen and release it with much less risk. Therefore, the aim of this exercise is to get as much movement as possible without stretching.

Do up to 10 repetitions and as long as it does not aggravate the symptoms the exercise can be done up to one set every 2 hours.

Acute low back pain

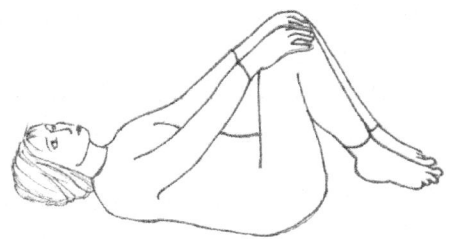

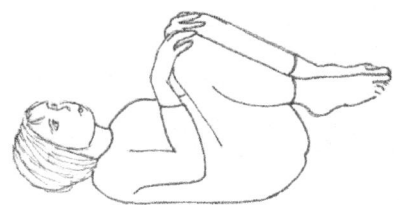

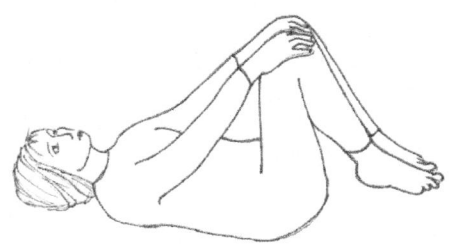

Exercise

Hip release exercise – good for low back pain and posture

This exercise gently releases and relaxes the hip joints. All the main muscle groups in the back have a strong connection to the hip joint. Therefore, releasing or relaxing the hip and associated muscles has a strong effect in relaxing the muscles in the low back.

The exercise involves feeling into the hip joint. By feeling into I mean focusing on the sensations produced in the hip joint as you move it and bring your weight onto it. Because this takes a bit of practice placing your hands over the hip joint will help you to focus on the area.

To start stand with your feet about the same distance apart as the length of one of your own feet, with the inside edges of the feet roughly parallel. Place one hand palm toward the body over the centre of the groin on the same side of the body (the hip joint is directly under this area). Then place the other hand behind the body and directly behind the position of the first hand, but with the back of the hand toward the body.

Slowly shift your body so that about 80% of your weight is over that hip. Then bring the weight slowly back to the middle again. Then slowly repeat. As the weight moves to one side this causes movement in the hip joint and alters where your weight is placed. Try and feel the effects of this in the joint. You may sense movement or change in pressure as the weight comes on and off the hip, try and focus on what is happening in the hip joint.

At first it can be quite difficult to feel anything. But if you continue to practice you will increase your sensitivity and be able to feel the hip working more easily.

Try a few repetitions on each side at intervals throughout the day. When you have low back pain standing still will often make the back tense up and feel worse. This exercise is useful because it can be done in many situations and enables you to avoid standing still.

Acute low back pain

If you have acute pain mainly on one side of the low back, be careful not to focus too much on doing this exercise on that hip. If you keep bringing your weight onto the injured part of the spine it may aggravate the injury. While your back is very painful on one side focus mainly on the opposite side. By doing the opposite side the whole back will benefit becoming looser and more relaxed.

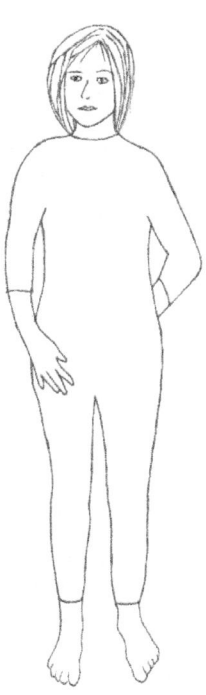

Acute low back pain in detail

Acute low back pain can be felt suddenly or build up over a few hours or days. Try not to panic. When people get back pain they tend to feel anxious and worry that it will not go away. Try not to worry as back pain normally settles on its own, and there are ways of helping to speed recovery. Most episodes of acute back pain are chance events due to a combination of factors that are difficult to predict or prevent. This kind of episode is only of concern if it starts happening regularly. If this is the case also read the next chapter, "recurrent low back pain".

When you have an acute episode of low back pain this normally means you have overworked some of the tissues that connect joints in the low back. These tissues become inflamed as a result of this damage. Inflammation is the production and release of chemical substances from the damaged tissues. Some of these chemicals are irritating to the area around the injury. This chemical irritation around the injury from inflammation often causes a large part of the pain felt after a low back strain, and is usually the cause of referred pain. Referred pain is where an injury causes pain to be felt in an uninjured area, in the case of a low back injury this is often the buttock or leg.

As a reaction to injury the body will try to protect or guard the injured area. This involves a tensing of the muscles around the injury and has the effect of reducing movement in the injured area. Initially this is not necessarily detrimental. In hospital for example when people have a bad rupture or fracture they will be immobilised in plaster. This is because if damaged tissue is moved or stressed too much it disrupts the healing process and prevents the damaged tissues knitting back together.

Managing acute low back pain

Avoid stretching too early

As mentioned earlier normally when you have back pain the back will also feel stiff. In trying to manage acute back pain people mistakenly assume the stiffness they feel around the injury is harmful and needs to be addressed. They often attempt to stretch away the tension in the muscles that are guarding the injury. This is of little help because the muscle tension is a reaction to the injury and not the injury itself. In the short term if you try to stretch this tension away the body will tense up again. Also during the initial few days when the injury is very inflamed pulling the joint around to stretch the muscles will often aggravate the injury.

Resting and gentle movement

For the majority of back pain injuries in the initial few days after the injury has occurred the best way to manage the problem is through a combination of rest and gentle movement. The most comfortable resting position for most types of acute low back pain is usually lying on the less painful side, knees slightly bent with a pillow between the knees, so the knees are separated by about 4 inches. If the pain is right across the back then lie on whichever side is more comfortable. If lying on the back is the most comfortable that is fine too.

Avoid lying on your front

However, avoid lying on your front even if it seems the most comfortable position. Lying on the front for any significant time will in the long term aggravate most types of back pain, even if seeming more comfortable in the short term. When you lie on your front the natural hollow or curve in the low back is increased causing the joints in the low back to be pulled out of their most relaxed position.

In very rare cases of back pain, people find lying on their front is the only comfortable position. If this applies to you I suggest you treat lying on your front as an exercise and do it for limited periods of 10 or 20 minutes combined with lying on your side or back. If you have to lie on your front put pillows under your stomach and pelvis, slightly raising this area by a few inches. This reduces the negative effect of lying on your front by reducing the hollowing effect on the low back.

Avoid the sitting position

Resting your back in a position with the least strain on the injured joint is vital to assist recovery. The position of least strain is lying on your side or back and gives the damaged tissues periods of reduced workload to repair themselves. As far as the joints in the low back are concerned sitting is quite a stressful position. It is stressful because firstly when sitting there is the same weight on the low back as in standing. Although we may feel we are resting when we sit because weight on the legs is removed, the joints in the low back continue to carry your upper body.

There is a second more subtle effect in sitting which then increases work for the low back joints. When sitting you bend the hip joints and as they bend into the sitting position they exert a pull through the muscles and ligaments on the pelvis and low back. This pull changes the shape of the low back so that the joints are no longer in the position of least strain. Due to these two effects most people with low back pain find the more they sit the longer the problem takes to resolve.

Encouraging gentle movement in the back – walking

In addition to resting the injury to give damaged tissues a chance to heal, movement is also important. Movement loosens the joints stopping them stiffening up. It also stimulates the flow of blood and fluids. This can help disperse inflammation and encourage healing. One of the best movements is walking which promotes gentle movement of the back and pelvic joints without strain. Walking is also a weight bearing exercise which is good for maintaining general fitness. If you have acute low back pain moving around the house or going for short walks interspersed with resting is a good way to start to improve your symptoms.

Please note, as mentioned in the last 2 pages, avoid resting in a sitting position or lying on your front. In these positions the back joints are under strain.

The correct way to get up from the lying down position

When people have acute back pain they often find lying down removes the weight on their back making the pain manageable. But when they sit or try and stand the pain becomes severe. The most common mistake is to try getting up from lying down and stopping half way, to rest in a sitting position. This makes the pain worse and may force you to lie down again. Although it causes some pain the best way to try and get up from lying down is to do it all in one movement, from lying on your side to standing.

To accomplish this move to the edge of the bed or sofa, while lying on your side facing outward. Let your legs swing down to the floor while at the same time pushing yourself up with your lower arm. Then try to come straight up into standing. If necessary get someone to help support you so you can achieve it without sitting half way. Once you are up don't stand still as this will make your back tense up. As soon as you are standing slowly walk about, and try to keep moving. If the pain starts to build up again or you feel you have done enough lie down again. When you lie down any increase in pain caused by standing up should start to subside fairly quickly.

If your back takes more than 15 minutes to calm down you have done too much. Next time you stand up and move around do so for a shorter duration. If however when you lie back down the pain calms down within one or two minutes, you know you can spend a little longer upright and moving about on your next attempt.

I have included some gentle exercises at the beginning of this chapter which are useful for people with acute low back pain, and can supplement walking around. If initially any upright position with weight on the spine is too painful, you can gently mobilise the back with a few repetitions of whichever of these exercises you can manage.

Use of medication to ease acute low back pain

Anti-inflammatory

Many of my patients prior to seeing me will have taken over the counter anti-inflammatory medication such as ibuprofen for their acute low back pain. My advice is to be aware that this type of medication can cause side effects for some people with common conditions such as asthma, hypertension and stomach or digestive problems. For example in about one third of people with asthma, anti-inflammatory drugs such as ibuprofen can make the condition worse. If you have asthma and are sensitive to ibuprofen the normal reaction is to start to wheeze within one or two hours of taking the medication. Fortunately for most people with asthma this reaction is mild and not life threatening. None the less for people with asthma who are sensitive to anti-inflammatories my advice is to avoid taking them. If you have any medical conditions and intend to use over the counter medication especially something you have not used before, it is advisable to check with the pharmacist before proceeding.

For most people taking ibuprofen is an obvious response to acute back pain. Ibuprofen is an anti-inflammatory and inflammation has a large part in causing the symptoms in acute low back pain. For this reason anti-inflammatory medication is recommended by most medical guidelines for treating acute low back pain.

Painkillers

For people who have acute low back pain painkillers may be helpful in the following situations.
Firstly, if you are unable to find relief in any position and having difficulty sleeping or resting, taking a painkiller may help.
Secondly, a painkiller may help people with back pain to attempt gentle activities such as walking. As mentioned previously moving

about carefully is helpful for people with back pain, because it can help to gently release tension and stimulate the injury in a positive way.

Studies confirm that people with acute back pain who initially rest for 2 or 3 days then despite the pain gently make themselves move about, will recover more quickly than those who continue to rest and are inactive.

Muscle relaxants

Muscle relaxants are another type of medication often used for back pain. However, some recent studies have found that muscle relaxants such as diazepam are not as helpful as previously assumed in treating back pain and may even have a negative effect on recovery. Muscle relaxants have a sedative effect, making people less active and less likely to make themselves move about if they are in pain. This tendency for muscle relaxants to make people more inert is assumed to be the reason why in some trials they have not always proven helpful in treating back pain. Although it could be argued that the sedative effect of muscle relaxants might be helpful in some instances, for example when taken at night to assist sleeping while in pain.

Medication - low success rate

Medication may seem the most convenient way to treat back pain, however a high percentage of back pain and other types of joint injury respond poorly to medication.

Therefore if your back pain does not respond to medication it does not mean your injury is necessarily unusual or life threatening.

The poor success of medication when used for back pain and many other types of joint injury explains why many people rely on chiropractors, physiotherapists and osteopaths to treat these conditions.

How long before you feel better

Carefully following the management approach in this chapter will have a helpful effect on most acute low back pain within a few days, particularly in people with no previous recent episodes.

If after 2 or 3 days there is no sign of improvement, a check up with a healthcare professional, such as your family doctor or someone who specialises in treating back pain, such as a chiropractor, physiotherapist or osteopath, is recommended.

If after a few days there is significant improvement in your back pain, this will tend to confirm that you are suffering from a simple back strain and that with care it will resolve without any need for treatment.

Sometimes however, back pain will initially start to improve but then the improvement stops and the symptoms fail to settle. If you continue to have significant discomfort after 2 or 3 weeks, even if you are able to perform most of your normal activities, it is advisable to seek treatment.

This is because statistically most low back pain that is going to settle without treatment has resolved or is well on the way to resolving after 3 weeks. There is a tendency in people who have significant back pain after three weeks for the back pain to continue long term if left untreated.

Chapter 2
Recurrent low back pain
(Persistent episodes of low back pain that returns within a few months)

What to do during a painful episode

Treat similar to acute low back pain, see chapter 1
Avoid sitting.
Avoid standing still
Move about or lie down.
If moving about eases the pain, include rest periods lying down.
Don't lie on your front. Lie on your side with a pillow between your knees or lie on your back.
Try not to do anything that aggravates the pain such as bending or lifting.
If lying down is the most comfortable position, when you can manage get up and walk about for periods as well, but avoid getting up and down every 5 minutes which jars the back.
If you can't find relief from pain in any position, making it difficult to sleep or relax, or if your symptoms are not improving within 2 or 3 days seek advice from a healthcare professional (see chapter 11).

What to do between episodes

Continue being careful between episodes, because you are not in pain does not mean the damaged tissue has fully healed.
Look at improving seating and working position to reduce the stress in your back, chapter 7
Improve posture, chapter 10
Do exercises to improve control and stamina of your back and pelvic muscles, chapter 3 & 12
Increase flexibility in the hip joints, chapter 12

Recurrent back pain in detail

Recurring back pain is when episodes of back pain initially settle, but within a few weeks or months return. This is of more concern than a single episode. Although recurring back pain is unlikely to be due to anything life threatening it is a sign the injured joints are not stabilising or healing properly between episodes. If not addressed this could lead to the back becoming more unstable and the back pain becoming constant.

With an episode of back pain of this type the first priority is to get the injury to calm down and reduce the pain. Initially it can be treated as in an acute problem, following the same advice as for acute back pain given in the previous chapter. In brief, avoid sitting and strenuous activity, have periods of gentle movement like walking as well as periods of rest lying or reclining, and seek help if the pain does not start to settle in a few days.

In my experience it is vital for those with recurrent back pain to remember that "**when it stops hurting it does not mean the injury has healed**".

To explain in more detail, most persistent or recurrent back pain involves damage to the discs or ligaments in the back. The discs and ligaments serve as bindings holding the back bones together, in exactly the way ropes can be used to hold things in place. Because vertebral discs and associated ligaments serve the same purpose as ropes in the body, holding things together, they don't need to be very biologically active to do their job (in the same way that rope is inert but it has a job to do).

Tissues, like ligaments in the body are not active and don't use much oxygen or energy. This means they don't require a good blood supply. How well and quickly any area of the body will heal after injury is generally proportional to its level of biological or metabolic activity. Because the ligaments and inter-vertebral discs that hold the spine together are not very active they are slow to heal. In common with ligaments in other areas of the body they can take many months to fully heal and strengthen after damage.

Taking your time: When the pain subsides avoid returning to your normal level of activity immediately.

In the body nerves and blood vessels tend to run together. An area with only a small blood supply will also have a low nerve supply making it relatively insensitive. This means ligaments and discs in the spinal joints, being relatively inactive tissue have a very poor nerve supply, making them not very pain sensitive. The effect of this lack of sensitivity can be that after an injury they become pain free long before they have fully healed.

In my experience a key cause of recurrent back pain is people resuming their normal level of activity too soon. Initially when their back hurts they tend to take care and do less so the pain subsides. People assume because it hurts less their back has healed and resume their normal level of activity.

However, with back injuries the level of pain is not always a good indication of healing. You may be feeling a lot better but the injury has not yet healed. This means returning to a normal level of activity can put more stress on the back joint than the weakened tissues can cope with. As a result the wound opens up again and the back pain returns.

The low back is a very active area, almost every movement or activity involves some level of strain on the low back. The fact that the low back has to cope with so much work during normal activity can mean the healing process is slower than other less active joints in the body. I normally tell patients with recurrent episodes of low back pain, to remember that **when the pain goes away the acute or inflammatory stage of the injury has resolved. This is the beginning of the healing process not the end.**

Reduce activities that stress the back for at least 6 to 8 weeks

My advice to patients with recurrent back pain is to reduce activities that particularly stress the back for a further 6 to 8 weeks after becoming pain free. This gives the damaged tissue time to heal and strengthen more fully so that when they return to normal levels of activity the injury is strong enough to cope with the stresses placed on it.

All current recommendations for treating low back pain suggest maintaining a level of physical activity. However, the type of activities undertaken must be chosen with care. This applies especially to recurrent or chronic back pain where the injured joints have usually become very sensitive. Maintaining a level of activity helps maintain mobility and stamina. However, exercise needs to be done in a way that minimises the stresses on the injured tissues, thus giving them the best chance to repair.

Guarding – how the body protects an injury

When you hold an injured joint in a stretched or strained position you are pulling and tearing at the damaged fibres. This is why with a badly torn ligament or tendon a cast or splint is used to immobilise the joint completely, which allows the injury to knit together. Even with less severe strains the body will instinctively try to immobilise the injury to reduce stress on the injured tissues. The way the body does this is to tense all the muscles around the injury to protect it. This is called guarding and is a normal reaction to injury. Unfortunately many people misinterpret guarding as the cause of the pain. For instance patients often say "I have had pain in my low back and buttock for several months. I know what's causing it because I can feel the muscles are tense so I have tried stretching and massage but I can't get the muscles to relax".

This is typical of someone with guarding due to an injury to one of the joints in the low back. Muscles are much more active metabolically than ligaments and other structural tissue and can heal within a few weeks. Therefore if a problem lasts more than a few weeks the source of the problem cannot normally be an injured muscle. If muscles keep tensing up in the way described by this patient, it is usually because the muscles are trying to protect something. With this type of injury people can inadvertently make things worse. The body is trying to immobilise the injured joint by tensing the muscles around it.

Stretching can delay healing

Like the patient mentioned many people incorrectly interpret the tension caused by guarding as being the source of their pain. They assume that if they release the tightness in the muscles the pain will go away. However, in most long-standing back pain muscles are not the primary source of the pain. The muscles tense because they are reacting to a stimulus from an injury underneath. As long as this injury exists the body will keep tensing up the overlying muscles. Trying to stretch in these cases has no lasting benefit in reducing the tension in the muscles, in fact quite the opposite. In these cases persistent stretching of the injured area stresses and irritates the injury which will increase muscle spasm and also delay healing.

Chronic back pain – mild low impact exercises

I advise patients with chronic back pain to do only mild, very low impact stretches, such as the legs against the wall exercise in the next chapter. To focus more on gentle mobilisation exercises such as those in chapter 1. Mobilisation exercises encourage improved movement of the joints without stress or strain. Patients with back pain who have been doing a lot of stretching find they improve once they apply a gentle approach, which does not involve strong stretching.

Activity – the negative and positive effects

People who are fairly active during the day and don't do much sitting, usually find their low back pain is at its minimum during the middle part of the day and worse in the morning or evening, or both. This is because activity during the day has both a positive and negative effect. Activity can have a negative effect on an injury due to the stress it causes to damaged tissues.

The positive effects of activity

However, physical activity also has a positive effect, the movement involved in everyday activity tends to loosen joints and stimulate movement of fluids that help disperse inflammation. It is because of these positive effects that back injuries can often feel at their best in the middle part of the day, when people have been moving about for a while. However the benefits of activity my not last all day. Often by the afternoon the injury starts to feel worse again as the stresses on it from prolonged activity start to have an impact.

Many patients want to know why their back feels worse when they have finish work and are resting at home. The answer is that when activity stops at the end of the day the positive effects of activity subside. Because the joints are not being moved, they start to tighten up and inflammation can build up. Despite this resting can be beneficial.

Resting reclined or lying encourages healing

When resting reclined or lying, you are taking weight and stress from the injured joints, which allows the damaged tissues to calm down and encourages healing. It is important to remember there are benefits to lying down even if it makes your back stiff and more painful. It is not lying down that makes your back worse it is just that it allows the symptoms to become more obvious and without some periods of rest the damaged tissues cannot heal. I would recommend if you are having an active day try to take 2 or 3 rest periods of at least 30-40 minutes each where you lie down or recline.

Protecting your back during the day

With long-standing back pain usually how stiff and sore your back is at the end of the day or the next morning, is proportional to how much you did to irritate it during the day. The more you protect your back during the day and minimise activities that stress the injured area, the less irritation and pain will surface when you rest and in the mornings on waking.

The benefits of walking

This tendency for the back to become stiffer after rest and in the mornings can lead people to think stretching their back at these times will help. But for someone with long-standing back pain this actually tends to irritate their back. As explained before, stiffness associated with chronic back pain is most likely caused by a guarding reaction, and not because there is something wrong with the muscles. If your back is stiff in the mornings you should get up, move around naturally or go for a walk. The back will ease even without specifically stretching. Stretching can be helpful but not for chronically irritable low back joints. Stretching should be avoided until any inflammation has settled and the irritability in the joints has stabilised.

Walking in moderation

Walking in moderation is a safe exercise. As with other exercises, a sensitive back will usually benefit more from several short walks than a single long one. If your back is very sensitive while walking you should avoid gradients. Walking up or down hills involves the body leaning forward or backward against the gradient. This puts extra strain on the low back joints and can irritate them if sensitive.

Acute pain – gentle exercise

The gentle exercises included in chapter 1 for treating acute back pain may be used. These exercises focus on mobilising the spine without stressing the joints and are usually safe to do even if there is some inflammation in the joints. However the maxim for exercising any part of the body that is sensitive and may be inflamed is "little and often" I normally suggest 10 repetitions of the exercises 3 or 4 times during the day. My advice is to do what is comfortable for you. If 10 repetitions seem to irritate the area then do less. For a very sensitive back start with just 5 repetitions.

After exercise if your back feels more painful and this extra level of soreness does not settle within about 15 minutes then you have done too much.

Prevention
What can you do between episodes to help prevent them?

Taking care of your back

Most injuries in the back or neck occur because these areas are under constant use. Therefore reducing their work load is vital to enable them to recover. This may be achieved by improving posture and the efficiency of your working situation. How to do this is explained in chapters 7 and 10. Over the course of a day by making changes to your posture and work station, the total stress put on an injury can be significantly reduced. This in itself may be enough to enable an injury to heal.

Exercise

Prescribing corrective exercises is not a simple matter due to the wide variety of lifestyles, occupations, age and fitness, which affect the degree of recovery and how individuals respond to specific exercises. Therefore, in difficult cases a professional practitioner will ensure an individual can be assessed taking into account factors such as lifestyle, age, body type, the nature of the injury and its severity. All these factors will influence the outcome of an exercise program. Taking into account these variables, I have suggested exercises my patients find effective and have safely applied for themselves. However, should problems arise I recommend an individual assessment from a professional practitioner. For more information about practitioners see chapter 11.

Using the exercises in this book to help restore natural movement in the back

Once we reach adulthood the hips become stiffer, which forces us to move more from the waist. If adults stop using the hips to carry most of the weight of bending and other movements and instead use the low back joints, it causes overload and injury. Once the low back joints are injured incorrect habits can slow down or prevent healing. For these reasons the exercises I have included for chronic low back pain in chapter 3 are aimed at increasing activity and stamina of low back stabilising muscles, and increasing hip flexibility. These exercises will have a significant effect in restoring natural movement to the back.

Increasing activity and stamina of low back stabilising muscles - good for natural movement

Around the spine in the area of the waist are several groups of muscles that help to stabilise the low back (lumbar spine). When the low back is under strain these muscles are activated. They not only reinforce the low back but also as they are activated and contract, have the effect of stiffening the waist area. This helps to prevent bending at the waist and overloading of the joints in the low back.

Increasing hip flexibility – good for natural movement

It follows that encouraging activity in the core muscles around the waist will stiffen and reinforce the spine when it is under strain. Also regaining flexibility in the hip joints will enable the body to start moving again from those joints, producing a more natural distribution of stress and protecting the low back.

Exercise – The do's and don'ts

Many people tend to believe that if they have an injured back they should do back strengthening exercises and stretching. In this section I will explain why this is incorrect and inadvisable.

Before undertaking any exercise a key question to ask yourself is how much exercise is the injured area subjected to during your normal life. The low back is an area that even during normal daily physical activities undergoes significant amounts of movement and stress. If you have maintained a normal level of activity and particularly if you have a physical job then your back should be reasonably strong. Therefore, to increase the strength of the back muscles significantly will require a lot of extra exercise. However, increased exercise increases strain on injured joints risking aggravating any injury.

Case Study

I interviewed a patient with a moderate, fairly constant ache in the low back which had persisted for several months. Three weeks after the onset he consulted a non specialist medical practitioner who advised stretching his back and to take up swimming. Despite following this advice the back pain continued. The patient worked as an electrician which is a highly physical job involving frequent stretching and bending and negotiating awkward, cramped spaces. On examination I found the ligaments between his lower back joints were sensitive indicating a strain in that area. I concluded that while there was no major structural damage, the workload being placed on the injured joints by the physical nature of his job was inhibiting their recovery. Moreover the recommended stretching and swimming was adding to the workload of the low back joints and slowing the healing process further.

I treated the injured area and suggested strategies he could use to help protect his low back from unnecessary strain. On my recommendation he stopped the swimming and stretching. Despite having his problem for many months, within a week his symptoms improved, and within three weeks the symptoms had gone completely. This demonstrates how too much exercise can inhibit healing of injured joints.

Exercises to increase low back strength and flexibility can be detrimental

Increasing low back flexibility is not recommended for chronic low back pain

There is no proven benefit to stretching a chronically injured low back. In fact quite the opposite. Studies have shown that people who have recurrent episodes of back pain, suffer more episodes if they exercise to make their back more flexible.

Any injured area of the body will normally feel stiff and tight. These feelings of tightness associated with injury will often cause people with back or neck pain to stretch the injured area. However, if we examine the activity involved in most people's daily lives we see a lot of movement and bending takes place in the low back and neck. When these areas are injured the body's normal response is to tense up around the injury to guard and protect it from further damage. Therefore, with back or neck pain the affected area is usually tight because the body is trying to protect the injury. This protective response is a neurological reaction and not the cause of the pain. Particularly in people with long-standing back problems trying to stretch tension away tends to work against the body's natural healing mechanism and aggravates the injury.

Loosening the hips and pelvis – good for chronic back pain

The hips are the strongest joints in the body with the largest muscle groups. Many of these muscle groups are also common to or connected to those in the low back. Therefore, increasing flexibility in the hips and pelvis has the effect of loosening and relaxing the low back, but can be done without placing much strain directly on injured low back joints.

Exercises to loosen the hips and pelvis

In chapters 3 and 12 I have included a number of exercises to help loosen the hips and pelvis. If you are using similar exercises make sure they have the effect of loosening the hip joints without putting much stretch through the low back.

Why you should avoid indiscriminate stretching of the low back.

Practitioners like myself will often stretch and loosen specific joints in the back as part of a treatment for a low back injury. This rebalances movement or releases compaction in joints. Professionals such as chiropractors, osteopaths and physiotherapists can do this in a way that minimises stress on injured tissue. It is very difficult to do this type of specific work on yourself, even for someone trained like myself. For the majority of those with chronic low back pain, indiscriminate stretching of the low back only aggravates their condition.

Increasing low back strength is not recommended for chronic back pain

To gain in strength you have to increase the size of your muscles. Muscles will only increase in size in reaction to high stress. It is easy to understand that exercising a damaged joint aggressively may not be helpful. If tissue is damaged it will become sensitive and inflamed. If you stress injured tissue too much it can inhibit healing. This is why bad joint injuries are immobilised with a bandage or cast.

When thinking about strengthening exercises we need to examine the kind of exercise to which your joints are normally subjected. For instance, in a job that involves a reasonable level of activity, your back joints are probably getting more exercise than you realise. Working the joints aggressively on top of this may mean the injured tissue is being overworked, which slows down the healing process.

Studies have shown that people with stronger back muscles are equally likely to suffer episodes of back pain, and during normal daily activity back muscles never use more than 10% of their strength. Therefore, if you have back pain and focus on aggressive back strengthening exercises, you risk making your condition worse with little benefit.

For back pain sufferers exercises for strengthening the back muscles are probably more appropriate for sports people or athletes who need a particular type of strength for their competitive activity. For most people I recommend gentle exercises which focus more on improving stamina and control and don't place stress on the low back joints. This approach has proved the most helpful to my patients.

Exercises to increase low back stamina and coordination are beneficial

Increasing coordination – good for low back pain

Doing any exercise repetitively will improve control and coordination. Repetitive exercise strengthens the nerve connections between the area being used, and the control centres in the brain, increasing the response of the muscles.

However, repetitive exercise will not necessarily increase muscle static strength unless it is done with significant force. Low to moderate impact exercises do not work muscles hard enough, or stress them sufficiently to stimulate muscle expansion. Gentle repetitive exercise can still be very beneficial, because it increases response in the muscles and can produce increased effective strength. For this reason exercises that produce gentle repetitive movements and muscle contractions can be used as the first phase of an exercise program for back injuries. They can be used to increase the effective muscle strength, without aggravating an injury that is in a sensitive state. Increase in control and coordination have also been shown to help prevent injury.

Increasing stamina – good for low back pain

It is essential to have enough stamina to be able to complete daily tasks and live an unrestricted life. If your pain is intermittent or manageable and allows you to carry on with most normal activities, then you will not be suffering with great loss of stamina. If however your activities have been greatly reduced due to pain, it is important to try to increase your activity level back toward normal to regain fitness. This may be achieved by increasing those activities which place least strain on the back joints. The most stressful activities for the back are those that hold the joints in a stretched position. That is a position where the back is being bent forward, backward, or twisted.

Exercises to avoid – those that hold the back in a stressed position

Bending forward, stretching forward.
Stretching the hamstrings/back of legs.
Any exercise from the sitting position e.g. cycling, rowing and any gym exercise done from the sitting position.
Bending backwards, lying on the front, sleeping on the front and any exercise done lying on the front e.g. swimming.
Any activity where the upper and lower body are not inline facing the same direction, or involves a lot of twisting movements.

How to increase stamina

Increase in stamina can be produced by intermittent, gentle to moderate exercise with rest periods. The exercise periods cause the muscles to adapt and increase stamina during the rest periods. The longer and stronger the exercise periods, the longer the rest periods have to be to allow muscle recovery and adaptation. If the rest periods are not sufficient for the amount of exercise, the muscles can degrade and less improvement is achieved. That is why trainers advise those doing strenuous exercise, such as running or weight training, not to train more than three times a week and to avoid training on consecutive days.

Low impact exercises to increase stamina – good for back pain

These are most exercises done standing up or lying on your back that do not jolt or jar your back. These types of exercise could include walking, stepping, cross training, free weights, pull down exercises (from standing) and bench press. I have also included some exercises in chapters 3 and 12 which help to increase stamina in the back. Take care to build up gradually from only a few repetitions if your back is sensitive.

For those with a history of back pain I especially recommend this low impact exercise regime for at least the first 6-8 weeks, to allow some settling and healing time after a painful episode. This can be frustrating because you may have to stop exercises you enjoy. As soon as you feel a little better you may be tempted to do the exercises I have suggested you avoid. However, the lack of pain you feel is not necessarily a reliable indication of the true state of recovery. Unless you are strict with yourself for a short time to allow proper healing your back may not heal properly and in the long term can produce more episodes of back pain.

Recurrent low back pain

Chapter 3
Exercises for recurrent or chronic low back pain

How to identify the best exercises for you

There are many different types of back injuries. Recovery from these injuries will not only depend on the nature of the injury and its severity but also a range of other factors such as lifestyle, occupation and any history of similar problems. Consequently, each individual with back pain will react slightly differently to exercise.

I have included exercises my patients have found the most useful and easiest to do. However, because it is difficult to predict how each person will respond I advise starting carefully. Begin by trying a few repetitions of each of the exercises recommended for your type of problem, then focus on four or five that seem the most beneficial. If your back is very sensitive limit your choice to one or two exercises. For those with very sensitive injuries doing a few repetitions several times a day is better than doing a lot all at once. This will help to minimise any painful reaction.

Muscle control/coordination exercises – good for back pain

Around the pelvis and trunk are muscles which help to stabilise the low back when it is under strain. Studies have shown that people with chronic low back pain have less active muscles in this region. This has given rise to the view that restoring lost muscle activity can help people with low back pain. This approach has become very popular in recent years and is widely used for treating low back pain, and is often known as the core stability method.

This approach is based on the assumption that when you exercise, if the muscles around the trunk and pelvis are poorly functioning they cannot perform their role in protecting the spinal joints. However, by the same logic this also means if you try to improve your muscles with aggressive exercises while they are still weak, the exercises may aggravate any back injury, as a result of lack of protection from those same muscles.

To avoid aggravating the injury I would advise patients with long term back pain to start with gentle muscle activation/control exercises. These are gentle exercises that serve the purpose of making the pelvic and trunk muscles more active. Making the muscle groups more active has the same impact as increasing their strength, because when your body needs to use these muscles to stabilise the back, it can activate the muscles quicker and more efficiently.

Simply put, the difference between the two approaches is as follows: **Strengthening exercises** use high force exercises to stimulate muscle cells to expand (not recommended for low back pain sufferers), whereas **activation/control exercises** use low force repetitive exercise to stimulate the nerve connections to the muscles (recommended for low back pain sufferers).

Despite their gentleness low force exercises if repeated enough, can have the effect of increasing muscle use and recruitment, but without the high stress associated with strengthening exercises. As a result there is a much reduced risk of irritating an injured area.

Activating the muscles – good for low back pain

Prior to suggesting exercises to increase stamina I normally show patients some gentle exercises to get their muscles to activate more fully. During these exercises you should feel your muscles contracting. Initially the contraction may feel slight. However, with persistence you will notice the feeling of contraction becomes more defined and that the contraction extends to more of the muscles around your pelvis. Sharpening the responses of these muscle groups will make them activate quicker and more completely and will in turn improve the way your low back joints are protected.

How many exercises should I do?

For people with long term low back pain it takes at least 6-8 weeks for muscle recruitment to show a significant improvement. This is achieved by using a regime of about 100 repetitions a day of one of the muscle contraction exercises, or a similar number of repetitions that combine some of these exercises.

Please note

To prevent the exercises aggravating chronic back pain avoid doing all of the repetitions in one session. I recommend dividing them into 3 or 4 sets of 25-35 with at least 2 hours between each set.

If you find doing 25 repetitions in one session aggravates your symptoms, start at 10 repetitions 2 or 3 times a day and over a number of days try to work up to 4 sets of 25 repetitions.

Exercises

Basic pelvic contraction – good for pelvic muscle activation

To start lie on a comfortable surface, bend your knees and bring your feet towards your bottom as far as you can comfortably.

Place your hands palm down by your sides and if you can push your fingers under the hollow of your low back, so the finger tips point towards each other and are 2-3 inches apart.

Without tensing or using too much effort, flatten the natural hollow in your low back by moving this part of your back toward the floor. Don't rush, take 2 or 3 seconds and relax, letting yourself follow the movement. This is important as the more you can follow the movement and control it, the more you are helping to strengthen the nerve connections to the muscles and increase their response.

At some point toward the end of the movement you may feel tension across the front of the pelvis. At the point when you start to feel some tension, do not go any further with the movement. Hold for 2 or 3 seconds then relax the back up again.

If you don't feel tension across the lower abdomen, which is contraction in some of the pelvic muscles, aim to go as far as you can without strain. Initially, if you cannot feel any contraction this indicates very poor muscle activity in the pelvis. There is no need to worry as this is not uncommon. Regular practice of this exercise you will bring improved muscle response across the front of the pelvis, as well as a response around the whole pelvis.

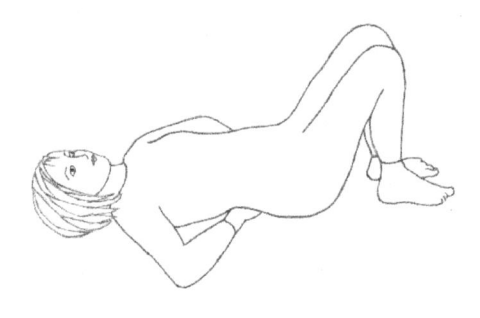

Exercise

Knee lift - good for pelvic muscle activation

This exercise causes a contraction in the pelvis and also has a mild strengthening effect.

Once you become used to doing the basic pelvic exercise, (pg 44) you can replace some repetitions of that exercise with the following to achieve an improved strengthening effect.

To start lie on a comfortable surface, bend your knees and bring your feet towards your bottom as far as you can comfortably.

Lift one knee up far enough so you can reach it easily with the hand on the same side.

Hold the knee in this position and gently push against it with your hand, feeling the contraction this causes in the pelvis.

Hold for a few seconds then replace your foot on the floor and relax.

Repeat on the opposite side.

This exercise can help to build stamina in the pelvic muscles that stabilise the low back.

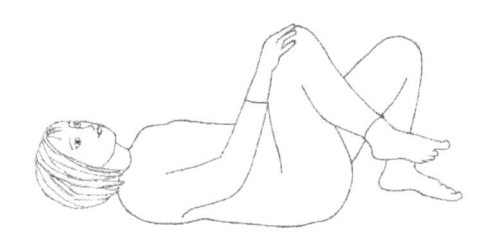

Exercise

Double knee lift – good for activating and building stamina in the pelvic muscles

To start lie on a comfortable surface, bend your knees and bring your heels up towards your bottom as far as you can comfortably.

Lift one knee towards your head, then bring the second knee up to join it. Hold in that position for a several seconds, then place the legs down again, one at a time.

With this exercise it is important to note that when you lift the second knee up into position, you may feel that your low back starts to arch up. If so you have not brought your knees up far enough. Bring your knees toward your head a little more until you feel your low back moving back to its natural shape. Hold the position for about 5 seconds.

Please note

If you have chronic back pain and your back is very sensitive leave this exercise (Double knee lift) until you feel able to achieve good contraction in the pelvis with the previous two exercises (pelvic contraction and knee lift). Even then I recommend introducing this exercise slowly starting with just a few and slowly building up to 10 or 15 repetition.

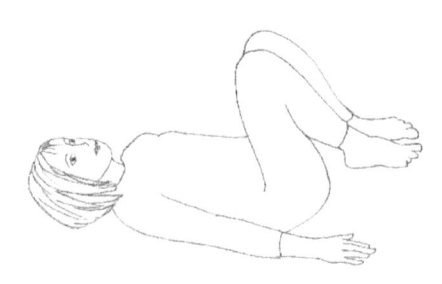

Further exercises to build stamina in the back and pelvis can be found in chapter 12.

Two Exercises for stretching the hips and pelvis – good for releasing tension in the back and encouraging natural bending

Many people with low back pain tend to assume that stretching their back by bending forward is helpful for their condition. However bending forward is usually very aggravating for people with a low back injury.

This is because bending forward from standing or sitting places a lot of stress on the low back joints and in particular on the discs. Therefore any stretching should be done cautiously.

The next two exercises done lying on the back produce a similar stretch to bending forward, but with reduced strain on the low back joints.

Please note
Both exercises should be tried carefully with awareness that they may aggravate back pain. Initially try the exercises gently for a short duration to explore their effects on your symptoms.

Exercise 1 Raised legs resting against a wall

To start lie on your back, raise both legs and place them vertically against a wall.

Pull your toes back and adjust your distance from the wall to get a comfortable stretch in the back of the legs.

Rest in this position for a few minutes, gently pulling your toes towards you to maintain a comfortable stretch in the backs of the legs.

This exercise is good for stretching the back of the legs, the buttocks and pelvis which releases tension in the back. For people with a sensitive back this exercise puts minimal stress on the low back joints.

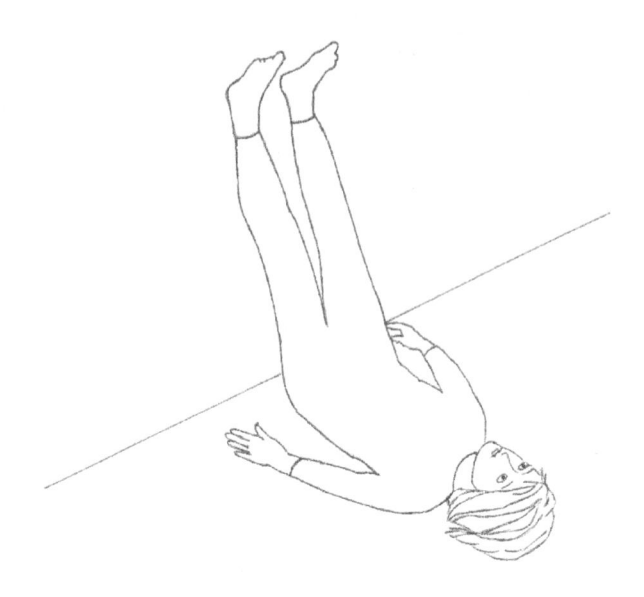

Modified exercise – raising one leg at a time
Good for people with low back pain.

The exercise above can be modified for those with a very sensitive low back injury by raising only one leg at a time.

To start raise one leg against the door frame of an open doorway while placing the other leg along the ground through the doorway. Continue the stretching action as in the previous exercise using one leg at a time.

The modified exercise produces less rotation and strain in the pelvis and lower back, and can be useful if those areas are very sensitive.

Exercises for recurrent or chronic low back pain

Exercise 2 Pelvis and hip stretch against a wall

With both legs raised and placed against the wall, let your knees bend and your feet slide down the wall as far as is comfortable.

Open your knees and allow the weight of your legs to stretch your knees apart until you feel a stretch in the hips and pelvis (this exercise also gives a good stretch to the knee joints).

This is a good stretch for the hip joints which has a powerful effect on loosening the low back.

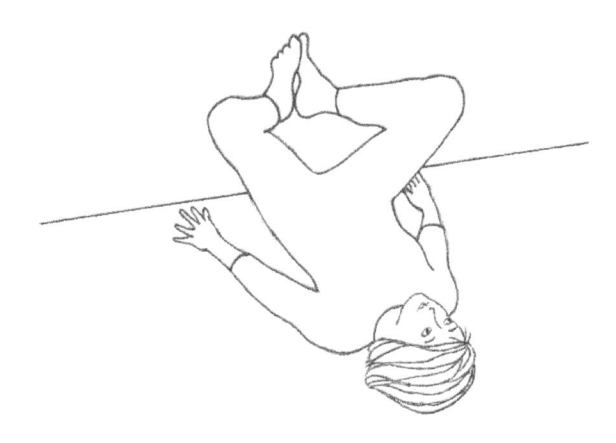

Further exercises to loosen the hip joints and pelvis can be found in chapters 10 and 12

Exercises for recurrent or chronic low back pain

Chapter 4
Sciatica

What causes sciatica?

The term sciatica derives from the sciatic nerve that runs from the low back into the back of the leg and is generally used to describe symptoms of pain down the back of the leg.

The term does not exactly define the cause of this pain, but is used if the source of the leg pain is thought to be a problem in the low back rather than the leg itself.

Back injuries can also give you pain in the groin and front of the thigh, though this is less common.

Symptoms of sciatica

If you have both back and leg pain then it is more apparent that your leg pain and low back pain may be connected. If you only have leg pain, there are several obvious signs that pain in the leg is likely to be coming from the back. For example if there is no sign of inflammation or other signs of injury in the leg, and when you touch the leg or move the knee or ankle joints, this does not make the pain worse. If in doubt consult a health professional.

There can be a number of causes of sciatica, most common is inflammation in the low back joints. Sometimes however, sciatica can be due to a more severe injury such as damage to an inter vertebral disc.

In general the further down the leg the pain is felt the more severe the injury.

Pain extending below the knee and into the calf or foot usually indicates some form of structural damage to a low back joint such as an inter-vertebral disc injury, often known as a slipped disc.

Slipped disc

A slipped disc is in fact not a disc that has slipped, but the term is commonly used to describe a damaged disc that has distorted enough to press physically on a nerve. This can cause pain down the nerve or if more severe can interfere with the function of the nerve. If pressure on the nerve is severe enough to affect its function the muscle or area connected to the nerve can feel numb or weak.

Foot drop

If the ankle feels weak enough to make it difficult to lift the toes during walking, this condition is known as foot drop.
Foot drop can be difficult to live with and can cause people to trip or fall resulting in injury. It should therefore be monitored closely.

If muscle weakness due to nerve compression is neglected, so that the nerve is subjected to a prolonged period of severe compression, the nerve may be permanently damaged leading to foot drop or other muscle weakness which may be irreversible.

The need for intervention – muscle weakness

When severe muscle weakness is not improving despite a few weeks of manual therapy there is a risk of permanent disability. Therefore, more invasive intervention may be necessary, such as an operation to release pressure on the nerve.

Loss of control of the bladder or bowel

Immediate intervention may be required if there are any signs that pressure on a nerve is causing interference with control of the bladder or bowel.
Loss of control of the bladder or bowel can have serious consequences and should not be left unattended.

When people with back or leg pain show any signs of change in bowel or bladder function an immediate MRI scan is required to fully assess the extent of the injury.

A back injury causing foot drop is rare and for a back injury to affect the bladder or bowel is even rarer. Most people with sciatica tend to suffer pain, sometimes with pins and needles or a small area of numbness, or both.

These cases will normally respond well to self help and the type of treatment provided by Chiropractors, Physiotherapists and Osteopaths.

Treating sciatic leg pain

Sciatica is most commonly caused by one of two conditions.
The first and most common is an inflamed joint in the spine. This irritates the sciatic nerve and produces leg pain due to inflammation infiltrating around the nerve. When this happens chemicals within the inflammation stimulate the nerve causing sensations of pain.

The second most common cause of sciatica is when damage to a joint in the back causes the joint to become distorted. This can lead to some part of the joint pressing on a nerve.

Distinguishing between these two conditions can prove difficult for the most experienced health professional. However, both can be grouped together for treatment. The treatment approach to these conditions largely depends on how sensitive or acute the injury is.

Acute sciatica

In cases where the joint is highly inflamed or sensitive the initial aim is to try and reduce the inflammation and sensitivity around the injury. This can produce improvement even if there is pressure on the nerve.
The most effective approach is to treat the injury in the same way as treating an acute low back injury that has no associated leg pain (see chapter 1). As with that type of injury the aim is to help disperse inflammation, gently restore normal movement to the joint, and use strategies to help protect the injured area from strain during daily activities.

Non Acute Sciatica

If the injury is not too irritable then more demanding exercises can sometimes help release a trapped nerve. A sign that a more demanding exercise approach may be possible is when the leg or foot pain does not change much during the day. That is, if the pain is not aggravated too much by most normal activities. This usually indicates that although there is pressure on the nerve the injury is not too inflamed.

In cases where the injury is not over sensitive, a successful approach devised by physiotherapist Robin Mackenzie, can be used. He found giving patients exercises which created repetitive movements in the area of the low back where a nerve was trapped would often improve their symptoms.

The success of these exercises may be due to a number of factors, such as the nature of the sciatic nerve which is a very thick, tough nerve, and the movement created by these exercises may enable the nerve to create space for itself by pushing any obstruction aside. Research also suggests that these exercises can help reduce internal pressure on a damaged section of disc.

Mackenzie's approach has been adopted world wide to treat patients with back and leg pain caused by disc injuries. However, it seems most effective if the disc is not too badly damaged or too sensitive and therefore may not always be appropriate.

Exercises

Knee rocking – good for acute and non-acute sciatica

To start lie on your back on a comfortable surface with your knees bent up and feet on the ground.
Lift one knee at a time then hold one in each hand with your arms straight and your knees together.
If your back feels stretched or uncomfortable in this position, avoid this exercise until it has improved. It is important to be able to hold this starting position without aggravating your symptoms.

Sciatica

If you are comfortably lying on your back you can continue the exercise. Rock your knees slowly towards your face. Use your arms to do this, not your leg muscles, so your back remains relaxed. At some point your low back will start to pull tight and begin to feel stretched.

As soon as you begin to feel the low back stretching, stop and pause for 1 or 2 seconds, then relax back to the starting position.

Please note: This exercise gently creates movement in the low back joints and is not a stretch. The injury may be very sensitive and if you keep stretching the damaged area you are likely to make it more inflamed and painful. However, if you use this exercise to repetitively move the joints without stretching, then you may be able to loosen and release them without irritation.

Try up to 10 repetitions and as long as it does not aggravate the symptoms the exercise can be done up to one set every 2 hours.

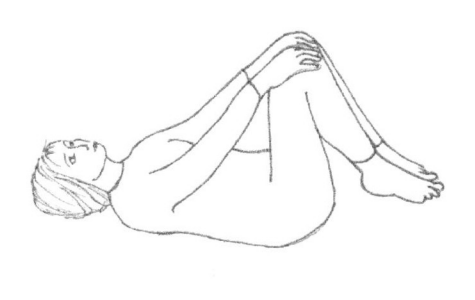

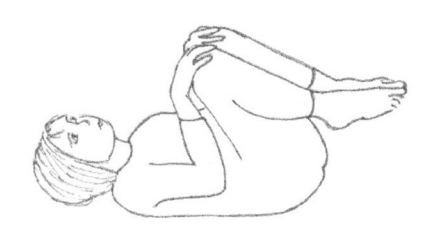

Side lean exercise – good for pain in one leg or pain in one side of the back

This is a good exercise if the sciatic pain is mainly in one leg. This exercise can also be helpful if the pain is felt in one side of the back without feeling leg pain. However, this exercise is demanding and can sometimes aggravate back or leg pain if the condition is very sensitive. Initially try 5 or 6 repetitions and if you find it helpful increase to 10 repetitions with a maximum of one set every 2 hours.

To start stand side on to a wall with your less painful side toward the wall and your feet together.
Position yourself and raise the arm nearest the wall until it is level with your shoulder and bend the elbow to 90 degrees.
Move yourself so that the elbow and forearm are about 8-10 inches from the wall.
Without moving your feet lean against the wall on your forearm. You should be near enough to the wall so this position is not a strain but far enough away so that when you relax your hips gravity causes them to drop naturally towards the wall without extra effort.
The exercise consists of gently relaxing your body so that the hips drop towards the wall, then straightening your body so that the hips come away from the wall again.

Please note:

This exercise is more demanding than it seems so do not push your hips towards the wall rather let them go as far as is natural helped by gravity.

Because you have the injured side away from the wall the exercise causes compression around the injury. This is thought to have a corrective effect on a distorted disc, as well as producing therapeutic movement in the joint

Doing the exercise the other way round with the injury towards the wall would not produce the same corrective effects and is more likely to cause irritation.

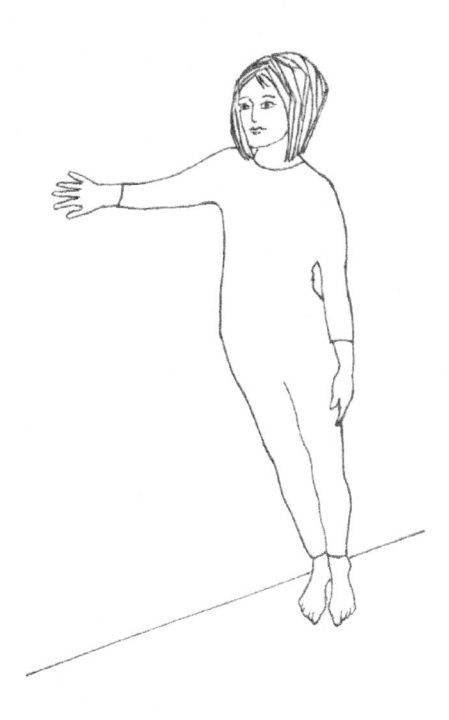

Sciatica

Exercise

Swinging knees to the side – good for age related stiffness and non-acute low back and leg pain

This is a good exercise for general age related back stiffness as well as for people with non-acute sciatica.

If your back is sensitive it is advisable to start with a few sets of 4 or 5 repetitions and assess if the exercise is helping or irritating your back. Low back injuries can be particularly sensitive to these kinds of twisting movements. Therefore, this exercise should be approached cautiously and may not be helpful if your back pain or sciatica is very sensitive.

If the exercise proves helpful build up to 10 repetitions in each set and several sets each day, with a maximum of one set every 2 hours

It is acceptable to continue doing less than 10 repetitions in each set if that feels comfortable.

To start lie on a comfortable surface with your knees bent up and together.

Swing both arms to one side then let your knees fall together to the opposite side, don't force your legs over to the side, let gravity pull them as far as they can go comfortably.

Relax in this position for a few seconds. Then swing the arms and legs together to their opposite sides. This can be a little awkward to co-ordinate at first but quickly becomes easier with practice.

Don't forget to pause and relax when your knees are over to the side.

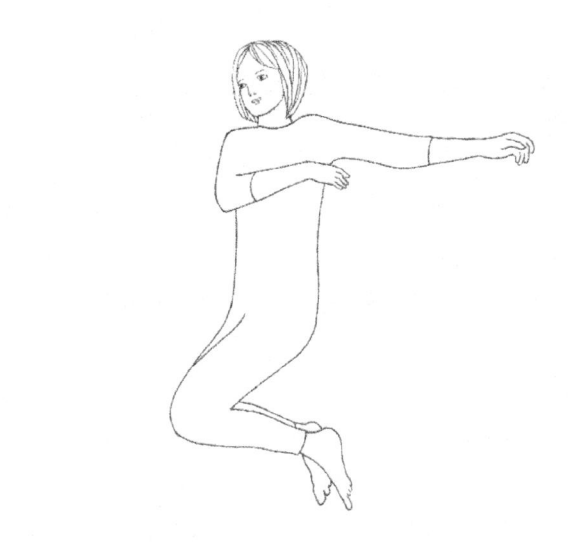

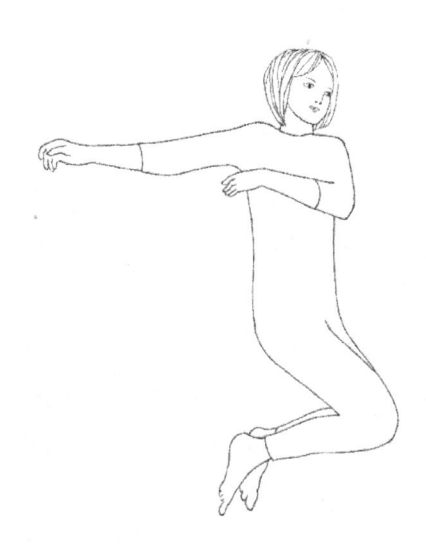

Sciatica

Exercise

Back extension - good for age related stiffness and non-acute low back and leg pain

This exercise is one of the most widely used for sciatic pain. As with the other exercises for sciatica the benefit of this exercise arises from the movement it produces and its effect on the disc, and not from focusing on it as a stretch.

I advise patients suffering from sciatica to start this exercise by placing some pillows or cushions under their pelvis, raising the bottom into the air. This start position has two benefits, firstly the back is more relaxed than lying flat on the stomach (which often aggravates sciatica) and secondly, this start position produces a bigger overall movement which can be beneficial.

To start lie face down on a comfortable surface. Place your hands palm down on the ground, just below your shoulders, fingers pointing forward.

Gently straighten your arms lifting your upper body off the ground but with your back relaxed so your hips remain down.

Go as far as you can comfortably or until you start to feel your hips lifting off the ground. Hold this position for a few seconds then relax back down onto the ground.

Pause and make sure you have let your body relax before you repeat the exercise.

During the exercise place your elbows into your sides, this keeps your shoulders down and your back more relaxed.

Please note:

With this exercise avoid using too much force which will place a lot of stress on the joints. This aggravates symptoms in a back injury that is acute and sensitive.

This exercise has the most benefit in cases of sciatica where the symptoms are not very sensitive and don't change much through the day.

Patients whose symptoms are aggravated by activity should approach this exercise cautiously starting gently with a few repetitions to gauge the effects.

Even if the exercise is helpful don't do more that ten repetitions in each set. If your back is sensitive do less. As with other exercises I have recommended, if your back is sensitive, exercise little and often.

Leave at least 2 hours between each set of exercises and reduce the amount of repetitions if your back starts to become more sensitive.

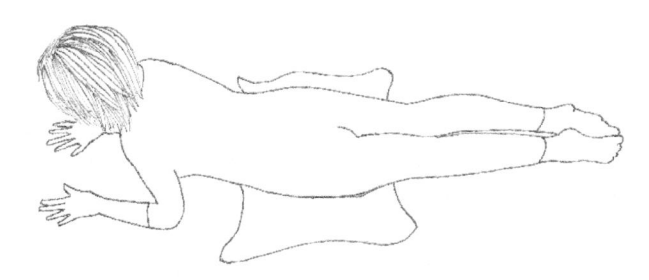

Sciatica

Chapter 5
Relieving long standing chronic back pain

Four stages in the treatment of longstanding back pain

Stage 1 The self-help route
Stage 2 Seeking help from a therapist
Stage 3 Further investigation
Stage 4 Pain management

Stage 1 The self-help route

Many patients have sought my help after enduring months or even years of back pain. In my experience long term back pain may be alleviated through self help. By following the self-help strategies I recommended, a significant number of my patients with long term back pain have achieved recovery.

The key self-help strategies are:

Identifying those activities which cause high stress and strain on the back. Modifying these activities or avoiding them altogether. How to do this is outlined in chapters 7 and 10

Increasing muscle control and stamina in the low back and related muscles, as outlined in chapter 3

Increasing flexibility in the hip joints, as outlined in chapters 3 & 12

These strategies are based on extensive work with patients who come to my surgery seeking help with a wide range of problems.

The direct and accessible nature of the regime I have devised for patients has had remarkable results in the relief of long standing chronic back pain.

Healing time: Time off work – increases the body's ability to heal

If you have a physical job or working situation which involves sitting all day, it may be not possible to change your work activities sufficiently to allow your back to heal. To reduce stress on your back and allow the back to improve it is advisable to remove yourself from the work situation.

During the time off work it is important to avoid bending, lifting or sitting for long periods. Reducing stress in this way can allow the back to start to improve. If you are receiving appropriate treatment from a therapist you may still need to take a break from work related strains to ensure your condition improves.

Stage 2 Seeking help from a therapist

It is never too late to seek help from a therapist. Osteopaths, Chiropractors and Physiotherapists often treat people who have chronic long-standing symptoms. It is not unusual for people to endure the misery of back pain for many months prior to seeking help.

Over 50% of patients treated by practitioners such as myself have had their problem for at least four months, and many have had their problem for a number of years.

As a result, Chiropractors, Osteopaths, and Physiotherapists are experienced in the treatment of long-standing problems. No matter how long you have suffered from back pain you will benefit from seeing a therapist.

Therapists and the treatment of back pain

More information about Physiotherapists, Chiropractors and Osteopaths, including approaches to the treatment of back pain and treatments used are given in chapter 11.

Stage 3 Further investigation

Chronic back pain can be very difficult to treat mainly because once the low back is injured it never gets a proper chance to heal as it is in constant use.

Further difficulty is caused by the lack of certainty in diagnosing the exact cause of back pain. X-rays are of limited use in difficult cases and MRI scans are not infallible.

Further investigation, when is it advisable?

The majority of back pain will respond to the types of treatment used by physiotherapists, chiropractors and osteopaths. If however, despite having treatment from a qualified therapist your problem persists, you will need to seek further investigation into the cause of your condition. This will normally take the form of an MRI scan.

MRI Scan

An MRI scan is more detailed than an x-ray and can show damage around the discs, soft tissues and the nerves. Further investigation using an MRI scanner will normally give enough information to suggest alternate treatment options.

However, MRI scans are not infallible as in some cases they are not able to locate the cause of back pain. In these cases additional investigation may need to be done.

Case Study

A woman in her thirties sought my help with disabling low back and leg pain. Over a period of five years her symptoms had gradually worsened, forcing her to give up work because she was unable to sit for very long, or walk very far without severe pain. She had previously undertaken a course of physical therapy, consulted an orthopaedic surgeon and had an MRI scan. The MRI scan showed nothing abnormal. The lack of findings on the MRI scan led the surgeon to diagnose chronic pain syndrome. Chronic pain syndrome is a situation that can occur when nerves have been registering pain over a long period causing them to become sensitised. The sensitised nerves will cause pain sensations even when the cause of the pain has resolved.

However, the patient was experiencing weakness and numbness in her leg, as well as pain. This is not normal in chronic pain syndrome and led me to query the diagnosis. I concluded that the condition was due to something pressing on the nerves into her leg. I subsequently referred the patient to a specialist spinal surgeon who agreed with my diagnosis that something was pressing on the nerves into the leg and causing the patient's symptoms. As a result he investigated further, in particular the area around the nerve roots in the spine, and discovered a small bony nodule pressing on a nerve. Once this was removed the patient made a full recovery and was able to return to work.

Seeking a second opinion

In the first investigation of this patient's complaint the necessary help was not forthcoming. The full range of possible diagnostic procedures were not undertaken and there was an over reliance on the MRI scan for a diagnosis.

Although the risks are low, there are more risks of complications occurring in surgery than other treatment options. Therefore, if a surgeon considers surgery unlikely to help a patient's complaint, they may not want to subject the patient to the risks of surgery.

However, not all specialists may be equally experienced in treating your particular condition. As in the case study above it can depend on finding the person most able to help you with your problem. I would recommend seeking a second opinion, particularly from someone who exclusively deals with your specific type of problem. For low back pain this would normally be a specialist spinal surgeon in one of the larger hospitals that have dedicated spinal units.

However, be aware that cases of back pain that require surgery are rare, more than 99.5% of patients with back pain will never need surgery.

Is seeking a second opinion advisable?

Many people feel that requesting a second opinion can be read as a criticism of their doctor which is not the case. Although back pain is not normally life threatening, the pain and disability it causes can have a profoundly detrimental effect on quality of life and mental health. My advice to those with a long standing problem is to explore all the options available to ensure the problem is investigated fully and to seek advice from the relevant professionals.

Specialist help, where to find it

I have devoted a section later in the book, see chapter 11, to treatments available for back and neck pain. If you have had treatment and found it unsuccessful, this section clarifies other treatments you can pursue.

Stage 4 Pain management

When self help proves ineffective in the relief of back pain the next step is to consult a therapist such as a chiropractor, physiotherapist or osteopath. Experienced therapists are able to draw upon a history of dealing with a wide range of patients and their problems.

Where a problem appears complicated the therapist will suggest a more thorough investigation such as using an MRI scanner. A scan will supply greater detail concerning the problem and increase the likelihood of a solution.

Occasionally surgery may be needed to correct a significant structural disturbance or instability.

Approaches to managing pain

In a small percentage of cases of back pain neither self help nor treatment proves effective. Furthermore, investigation proves unsuccessful in finding any physical cause for the pain or else indicates that treatment is not possible.

At this stage the emphasis is on pain management and controlling the symptoms in order to make the individual's life more comfortable.

Use of painkillers

There are several approaches to pain management, for instance the use of various types of common painkillers, such as those based on codeine. Alternatively, many people with chronic pain are prescribed drugs that were originally developed as anti-convulsants or anti-depressants. These are drugs such as Gabapentin, Pregabalin and Amitriptyline. There is little understanding of how these drugs help people with chronic pain but some studies have shown them to be useful. However, long term use of any drugs brings the risk of side effects.

Use of implants to control pain

As an alternative to high doses of painkillers, centres for pain management have introduced the use of devices planted inside the body to control pain. There are two types of device which are as follows:

Spinal cord stimulation

In spinal cord stimulation therapy a small device is implanted with two wires that send electrical impulses to the spinal cord. For reasons that cannot be fully explained, electrical pulses on the surface of the spinal cord can significantly reduce pain. Electrical spinal cord simulators can therefore be used to give relief for people suffering chronic pain. The advantage for patients is that they are able to control the stimulator using a remote control.

Implanted pump

The other type of implantable device used is a small pump which delivers painkillers to specific areas of the spine. By surgically implanting a pump under the skin, a tube from the pump can be placed to carry medication to a precise location in the spine. As the drugs can be administered much more specifically, much smaller doses need to be used compared to tablets or injections, this therefore can have a great impact on reducing side effects.

Psychological approaches to pain management.

Cognitive behavioural therapy (CBT)

Another method that seeks to move away from high levels of drugs to control pain is the use of psychological centred approaches. Of these, cognitive behavioural therapy (CBT) is the most widely recognised, based on the premise that ways of thinking have an impact on feelings and wellbeing.

Studies show that negative thoughts tend to heighten feelings of pain. CBT teaches techniques which help people to recognise when they are falling into negative thought patterns and gives them strategies for developing healthier, more positive ones. Teaching people to think and feel more positive has been shown to help people relax, feel less anxious, and reduce pain.

Using visualisation to relieve pain and tiredness

Visualisation is widely used as a means of controlling the feelings of tiredness and anxiety associated with pain. Although associated with eastern practises such as mediation, visualisation techniques are becoming more mainstream in western society.

Most people will be aware that visualisation consists of imagining a particular object or place. Many people may have tried relaxing using a visualisation CD or joined a yoga class where teachers often use visualisation to help relaxation.

As visualisation techniques are relatively easy to follow I have included exercises which can be tried at home

In visualisation the aim is to imagine a situation that produces a pleasant, enjoyable feeling. For example, on a cold, wet day imagine being in a place bathed in sunlight.

Visualisation works because although these things are imagined, to some extent the mind and body will react to them as if they were real. Therefore it is important when visualising to choose a situation or object which you know will make you feel comfortable, relaxed and positive. For instance, relaxing on a beach or in a garden, or imagining the feeling of sunlight on your body. Alternatively a happy memory, or anticipating a pleasant event such as a holiday.

Visualisation is most effective when you choose something to visualise that helps you relax and feel positive.

Relaxation technique combining visualisation and breathing

You will find guidelines to breathing techniques in chapter 10.
Once you feel comfortable focusing on your breathing you can try the following exercise which combines breathing practice with visualisation. Using this combination can make the relaxation effect more powerful.

Visualisation and breathing exercise

When you breathe in, if you are conscious of your breathing then your attention naturally follows the breath into the body. Likewise when you breathe out your attention follows the breath out of the body.

As you breathe in relax and let your attention follow the air entering your body. Imagine the air entering your body has a pleasant quality or is sweeping a positive, healthy feeling into your body. As you breathe in imagine this pleasant feeling moving with the breath into the centre of the body and down into the lower abdomen.

As you breath out your attention will naturally follow the air out of your body. Imagine as you breathe out that the pleasant feeling which came with the breath into the centre of the body and down into the lower abdomen, now moves outwards.

This exercise can be done any time throughout the day preferably in a quiet situation where you can concentrate.

Relieving long standing chronic back pain

Chapter 6
The common causes of back and neck pain

When you have back or neck pain it can feel as if the pain is never going to stop and as a result people imagine all sorts of causes for the pain. It may be comforting to know that the real cause is usually much less worrying than what you imagined.

In this chapter I will help dispel anxiety by providing information on the common causes of back and neck problems.

Anatomy of the spine

The spine consists of a column of blocks of bone separated by flexible washers which allow each bone segment to move with its neighbour. The bones are called vertebra and the flexible washers between are known as inter-vertebral discs. Immediately around this column are ligaments which bind everything together, and outside of this are muscles which can contract to pull on the spine. Muscle pull sometimes acts to hold the spine in position and sometimes to produce movement.

For medical purposes the back and spine are divided into three sections.

Thoracic spine
The middle section of the spine is defined as the area where each vertebra has a rib attached to each side. Normally there are twelve of these. This middle section of the spine is known as the thoracic spine.

Cervical spine
Above the thoracic spine there are seven vertebra without ribs attached. This forms the neck, also known as the cervical spine.

Lumbar spine
Below the thoracic spine there are also vertebra without ribs attached. This area is known as the lumbar spine or lower back, and normally consists of five vertebra.

Variations in spine structure

This in its simplest form is the basic structure of the spine. However, not all backs are exactly like this. A significant percentage of people may have some variation from this average structure.

These variations can include fewer or extra vertebra or ribs. Sometimes vertebra can be jointed together so there is no disc in between. Sometimes the bones are not formed in the correct shape. If the vertebra are not formed in the correct shape, the spine may curve to one side, a condition known as scoliosis.

In the past if an individual had one of these variations it would be seen as the cause of any back or neck pain the person may suffer. However, recent studies have shown that almost all genetic variations in the structure of the spine, including mild scoliosis, have much less impact on causing back pain than was first thought.

Most studies show that people with these structural differences do not experience more back pain than the average person, and if they do get back pain they are just as likely to respond to treatment. If you have been told you have one of these types of variation in the structure of your spine there is usually no cause for concern.

Back and neck pain – where does it come from?

Ageing – its effect on back and neck pain

There is a common misconception that as you get older back pain is inevitable due to wear and tear of the back joints. Any adult x-ray will indicate signs of wear and tear to the spinal joints even in people who have never had back pain. Wear and tear of the joints in the back is a normal part of the ageing process and in most people will not cause chronic back pain.

Contrary to popular belief the occurrence of low back pain in adults does not change much with age. In any year about 15% of adults will get back pain. This figure is approximately the same across all ages. This is because most back pain is not caused by obvious wear and tear of the bones but by other more subtle injuries.

Muscles Injuries

The spinal joints are shaped so that each bone in the spine makes contact with the one above and below at three points. These points of contact are the inter-vertebral disc at the front and two smaller joints at the back known as facet joints. The joints are strapped together by ligaments. On the outside of this are the back muscles.

The muscles have an active role in contracting to cause movement in the back and stabilise the back when it is under strain. Because the muscles are constantly working they have to have a good supply of blood to provide a high level of oxygen and nutrient.

As far as injuries are concerned one benefit of this high level of activity is that muscle injuries tend to heal quickly, usually within a few weeks.

Therefore if you have pain that fails to improve after a month, the cause is unlikely to be an injury of the muscles.

Ligaments and inter-vertebral disc injuries

Underneath the muscles are the ligaments and the inter-vertebral discs. Unlike muscles the ligaments and discs do not have an active function, they simply bind the bones together and help give strength to the joint. They are like the rope used to make a raft, performing a function without having to move or be active in any way.

Because ligaments and discs are not active, they only need to have a limited blood supply and very low level of biological activity. Consequently, if ligaments or inter-vertebral discs are injured, they can be very slow to heal. Any injury to ligaments can often take several months to heal and injuries to a disc can sometimes take longer.

How disc injuries cause pain

The inter-vertebral disc is a kind of circular ligament which is fibrous in nature. These fibres can become damaged causing the disc to become weakened and sometimes to distort. If the disc becomes severely distorted it can interfere with other structures that lie close to it. Though not a very exact description, the term "slipped disc" is often used to describe a disc that has become damaged and distorted enough to press on nerves close to it.

Pain from the sciatic nerve

There are two main nerves that can be affected by a slipped disc. The most commonly affected of these is the sciatic nerve. When the sciatic nerve is affected, pain is felt down the back of the leg and can also occur in the foot, ankle and lower leg. Because these types of symptoms come from the sciatic nerve this condition is often called sciatica, which describes pain coming from some form of irritation to the sciatic nerve.

The femoral nerve

The second nerve in the back that can be affected by a disc injury but much less commonly, is the femoral nerve. If this nerve is affected it can cause pain in the groin, front of the thigh and knee.

Pressure on a nerve

Pressure on a nerve due to a slipped disc can cause not only pain but other symptoms including feelings of numbness and also muscle weakness. In very rare cases, severe pressure on the nerve can affect control of the bladder or bowel. This leads to frequently wanting to go to the toilet or loss of control. Because of possible long term complications, interference with bladder or bowel control is considered a medical emergency. Immediate medical attention should be sought.

How damage to the disc occurs

Damage to the disc is thought to occur in one of two main ways. Firstly, due to repetitive stressing of the fibres of the disc causing a build up of fine tears. These small tears can then gradually join together forming a larger area of damage. Areas of damage on the disc cause weaknesses in the disc structure that eventually leads to the disc becoming distorted or rupturing more completely.

The second main cause of damage to discs is the result of a knock-on effect from damage to the bones in the spine that are above and below each disc. This is thought to be produced by a sudden jolt to the spine for instance, jumping off of a high wall. This can cause small fractures in the bone adjacent to the disc. At the time it occurs this injury may either not be noticed or seem very severe.

It is believed that if this type of small fractures in the ends of the vertebra occur, they can release small amounts of blood which infiltrate into the disc. As the disc does not normally come into contact with blood it is thought that this blood actually damages the disc, making it vulnerable to injury.

Some recent studies have also suggested that in some people these small fractures in the vertebra can become the site of a low grade chronic infection that can be the cause of back pain.

Damaged discs in long standing back pain

Damage to the disc is a common cause of long-standing back pain. This damage is sometimes obvious and at other times subtle. Major disturbance to the disc can usually be located easily using an MRI scan. However, small areas of damage to the disc can also produce high levels of pain. These small areas may be difficult to locate and may not be detected from an MRI scan.

Discography – detects damaged disc tissue

An alternative means of detecting areas of inflamed, damaged disc tissue is through the use of discography. In this procedure anaesthetic is injected into the area of suspected damage. If the tissue has become sensitised then an anaesthetic will temporarily reduce any symptoms. If the tissue is normal then no reaction will be felt. In chronic back pain areas of subtle damage to the disc can often be more significant than more obvious signs. A disc does not have to be pressing on a nerve to cause pain. Pain can also be due to inflammation from a damaged disc. During inflammation damaged cells within the injured area cause the release of chemical substances, many of which can irritate nerves, causing symptoms along the nerve similar to nerve compression. In rare cases where a disc is not pressing on a nerve its removal may still be necessary because it has become chronically inflamed.

To summarise, pain from the disc occurs in the following ways:

Small tears in the fibres of the disc can cause an area of sensitivity and inflammation.
Sometimes areas of weakness in the disc become unstable and distort, bulging out.
In severe form the area of bulging disc can distort further and press on a nerve. This is often called a slipped disc or a disc prolapse.
If the disc is in the low back then pressure on the nerves is commonly felt as pain in the leg and foot. These symptoms are frequently known as sciatica.
Even in milder forms of disc injury where there is no pressure on the nerve pain can be provoked in the nerves due to inflammation.

How facet joints cause back and neck pain

The facet joints are two small joints behind the disc that help stabilise the spine. Pain in this area can be caused in several ways. When the disc in front of these joints becomes worn or damaged it tends to become thinner. This loss of height in the disc can throw more pressure on the facet joints, increasing wear of the joints and causing them to become painful. Facet joints can however, cope with a lot of wear without causing problems. X-ray findings of facet joint wear are common in people with no back pain as are findings of reduced disc height.

Facet joint strain

A common cause of pain from the facet joints is due to over stressing of the joint, causing tearing of the surrounding ligament fibres. When this happens pain is felt and the overlying muscles will tense up to help protect the injury from further damage. If the damage to the ligaments is severe this can lead to the joint becoming weakened and unstable. Even less severe damage to the facet joint ligaments can lead to long term pain. This occurs because damaged ligaments often shorten and contract as they heal. If this happens the joints will not move properly and the ligaments are left in a state of abnormal tension. This is why some simple strains will seem to linger and refuse to heal without treatment.

Facet joint pain due to insufficient exercise or poor posture

Pain caused by abnormal tension around a joint can occur without any injury taking place. Joint tension can come on quite gradually due to lack of exercise or poor posture which leads to a gradual loss of movement in some areas of the body. Similar to what happens following an injury there is the same type of shortening and contraction in the soft tissue. This type of back pain related to postural tension most frequently occurs in the middle and upper back. For instance certain occupations such as working at a PC or driving, can cause both these areas to be held immobile for long periods.

How sacroiliac joints cause back pain

The sacroiliac joints are just below and on either side of the base of the spine. As with other joints, the fibres holding the joint together can become strained due to over stressing, and occasionally after a strain there is residual disturbance which causes pain.

Injuries in the low back joints will often be felt as pain around the sacroiliac joint and in the buttocks, due to referred pain. Pain can also be felt in the sacroiliac area due to problems in the muscles that support the low back, some of which are attached around the sacroiliac joints. This makes diagnosing sacroiliac injuries difficult as injuries to the spine will also cause pain and muscle spasm in the buttocks and around the sacroiliac joints. For example, patients will often believe they are suffering with a sacroiliac strain but following examination the cause of the problem is found in their spine.

Factors that slow recovery in ligament and disc injuries

In the low back the slowness of the natural healing rate of ligaments and discs can be exacerbated by the fact that they are subjected to continuous strain. Almost any movement of the body will tend to cause some stress in the low back (ask anyone suffering from acute back pain). The structures of the low back are being continually stressed throughout the day.

Slowness in healing of ligaments and discs combined with the continual work endured by the low back joints, can make recovery from relatively small injuries difficult, particularly if your work situation involves a lot of strain on the low back.

Because muscles are quick to heal and ligaments and discs very slow, chronic low back pain is most likely to come from damage to the core structural components of the back. These are the ligaments that hold the bones of the back together, the facet joints and intervertebral discs.

Osteoarthritis

Sensitivity caused by osteoarthritis can also lead to joints becoming tense which will exacerbate the symptoms. Exercises or treatment to help maintain movement and keep joints relaxed will usually help control the symptoms of osteoarthritis.

Can being overweight cause back pain?

A frequently asked question from patients with back pain concerns weight. For example, "I suppose losing a few pounds would help?" Despite numerous studies on the subject, there is no evidence that being overweight increases susceptibility to back pain. These studies correspond with my experience with patients who may be overweight but do not respond any differently to treatment. Neither do they need more treatment than patients of average or below average weight.

Although being overweight has been proven to contribute to other health problems, it does not seem to have a significant effect on back pain.

X-rays

X-rays are frequently used as a screening device for patients with back pain. However in most cases, the general state of wear and tear visible on x-ray taken after an injury will be no different from an X-ray taken immediately before. An X-ray can be useful in detecting fractures and other damage to the bones, but for the nerves, ligaments or discs, an X-ray gives no detail.

MRI scan

Therefore, it is normal practice for people with back or neck pain that is not improving or responding to treatment, to be given an MRI scan. This ensures a more thorough investigation of the symptom. An MRI scanner uses magnetic fields rather than X-rays and gives a much more detailed picture of the nerves and other tissues such as the discs and ligaments.

The common causes of back and neck pain

Chapter 7
Making changes to work and other daily activities

Studies have shown that modifications to the work situation and changes to daily activities relieve long term back or neck pain.
The following section outlines the changes which will help in the relief of back and neck pain.

Reducing sitting – good for relieving back pain

It is commonly assumed that sitting is a position of rest. Because sitting removes weight from the legs it makes us feel we are using less effort compared to standing. However, the sitting posture has been shown to significantly increase strain on the low back compared to being upright. This is due to the following, firstly in the sitting position the back continues to support the same weight of the upper body as it does standing. Secondly, the structure of the muscles and ligaments that connect the hips, pelvis and low back is such that as you sit, rotation of the hip joints exerts a pull on the joints in the low back. This causes the natural inward curve of the low back to flatten out, pulling the back joints out of their natural relaxed position. The lower you sit the more strain is put on the joints in the low back due to increased rotation of the hip joints.

Using the reclining or lying position – good for relieving back pain

When resting to ensure relief from back pain rest in a reclined or lying position which will transfer strain away from the low back joints.

How to adjust an office chair – good for back and neck pain

Adjusting the seat platform

If you are sitting upright in a working position, the seat platform needs to be tilted forward so the front is approximately 2 inches lower than the back but continues to feel comfortable and stable when you sit on it. You can locate this position by increasing the tilt until you find the point where you no longer feel stable. Then reducing the tilt slightly from this position so that you feel comfortable again.

Using a pillow or wedge cushion

If your seat cannot be adjusted then a large cushion or pillow can be placed across the back of the seat to achieve the same effect. Alternatively, an inexpensive wedge cushion can be obtained from an orthopaedic supplier, the internet, or your therapist.

Achieving the correct seat height

The seat height should be adjusted so that when your feet are on the ground the lower part of your legs below the knee are vertical. If your chair cannot be adjusted so it is low enough to achieve this posture then you can use a box or foot rest. It is best to avoid having your legs hanging in space as this will create a pull into the pelvis.

Adjusting the seat back

Because we are used to sitting supported, when we sit on a stool or seat without a back for more than 20 minutes, we tend to slump or collapse. If you have a seat with an adjustable back rest, placing the lumber support in the right place helps maximise the support given by the back of the seat. On seats with an adjustable lumbar support it should be placed at the centre of the hollow in the low back, which is roughly at waist level.

To find this point adopt a standing position then place a finger at the deepest part of the hollow in your low back. Keep your finger in that position as you sit down. This is where the middle of the lumbar support should be placed.

You should position yourself on the seat so that you are sitting upright, supporting your own back, with the lumbar support just touching the hollow of your back. Positioned correctly the lumbar support will prevent any tendency to collapse. However it should not press on your back hard enough to push the natural curve in your low back out of shape.

High quality chairs have seat platforms which can slide forward or backward relative to the position of the lumber support. If yours does not have this facility you can simply move yourself forward or backward on the seat to achieve the same result.

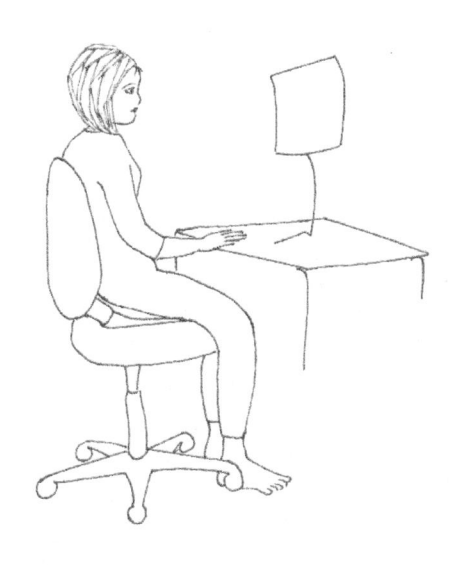

Adjusting the computer screen

Once the seat is at the correct height, adjust the screen of your computer so that your eyes are level with a point about one quarter of the way down.

If the screen is too high you will be looking slightly upwards which places stress on your neck.

If the screen is too low so you are looking downwards, stress is placed on your neck and tends to pull the posture forward and out of balance.

If your screen cannot be adjusted there are adjustable height stands especially for computer screens, alternatively books or reams of paper can be placed under it.

Achieving the correct desk height

The height of your desk is correct when your hands are working at the key board with approximately a right angle bend at the elbow.

If the desk is too low then you will have to reach for the keyboard which creates strain and pulls the posture forward.
If the desk is too high then you will have to use unnecessary effort in the arms and shoulders to hold the arms in a raised position.

Raising your desk

Well designed desks have adjustable legs. If the legs cannot be adjusted and the desk is too low, it can be raised by placing blocks under the legs.

Raising yourself

If the desk is too high it may be impractical to cut the legs down in which case your seat can be raised into the correct position. A box or foot stool placed under your feet will ensure your feet are supported.

Case Study

During consultation with a patient suffering long-standing chronic low back pain it emerged that he spent many hours a day sitting in front of a computer screen. We discussed how his incorrect sitting posture caused strain on his back which could be helped by using a fully adjustable chair. Following my advice the patient obtained the recommended type of chair from a specialist supplier. After only three days of using the adjustable chair at work he felt significant improvement in his comfort level. Within a few weeks any back pain he experienced at work was negligible.

Studies have shown that one of the most effective ways of helping people with long term back pain is through changes to their work activities.

Using an adjustable lumbar support in the car

In a car seat the lumbar support is meant to support the low back in the position of minimum strain (slightly curved inward). Adjusting the lumbar support so it is too far out should be avoided as it pushes your back into a distorted shape.

Kneeling stools – use for no more than 20 minutes at a time

When using a kneeling stool or other chair without a lumbar support sitting time should be limited to no more than 20 minutes. Most people find it difficult to maintain good posture for longer than this without support for their back. Another disadvantage with kneeling chairs is that to stop you sliding forward out of the seat they exert pressure on the knees. This pressure on the knees if sustained for a long period often leads to significant discomfort.

Positioning laptops correctly

Laptops or notebooks are commonly used at work and in the home. However the position of laptop screens are too low, even when placed on a desk. The low position of the laptop screen causes your head to drop forward as you look at it. This puts great stress on

Making changes to work and other daily activities

your neck and pulls your posture forward. An inexpensive solution is to use a separate keyboard and mouse. Using a separate keyboard and mouse with your laptop allows you to place the laptop on top of something to support it in the correct position, with the screen level with your eyes. This will remove a lot of strain from your posture, particularly your neck.

Avoiding sitting

No matter how good the sitting posture, sitting will always puts more stress on your low back compared with walking upright. As explained earlier sitting distorts the position of the joints in the low back therefore, most low back problems are aggravated by sitting. This is usually apparent to people with low back problems. However with some low back problems the irritation produced by sitting is not immediately obvious. For this reason sitting is best avoided even if it does not appear to make your back pain feel worse. For low back pain, the less you sit the quicker the problem will settle.

How to reduce the negative effects caused by sitting

Having a correct working position

If your work involves a lot of sitting you can minimise the stress on your low back by setting up your working position correctly, as described earlier in this chapter. Taking regular breaks from sitting by standing up and walking about is also recommended. Try to do tasks while walking about, for instance, telephone calls, drinking coffee or reading documents. If it is not necessary to sit at work, try to keep moving and remain upright rather than sitting.

Taking a break

During your work breaks walk about, being on your feet moving about rather than sitting is less irritating for low back pain. If you want to take the weight off your legs or pause for a snack, perch on a window ledge or table so that your hips are above your knees, and your thighs are sloping downward. This places less strain on your back compared to sitting in a low chair.

Resting in the correct position

Be aware that spending the whole day either standing or sitting, entails continuous working of the joints in the back. This is not an ideal situation for anyone with an injured back. For those people whose job entails long periods of standing or sitting I recommend taking a few breaks in the day to rest the back by lying down. If this is not possible during the working day try and rest your back as soon as you get home, before undertaking any activities.

The resting position is where there is minimal strain on the low back joints, ideally lying on your back, on your side or lying reclined. Lying on your front does not remove strain from the low back and neck joints and should be avoided.

The rest periods should be of at least thirty to forty minutes. A five or ten minute rest will be of little benefit to painful back joints.

If you suffer from back pain avoid relaxing in a sitting position during non-work time. For reading or watching television a reclined position can be more comfortable than lying down. Both lying and reclining are better than sitting because they reduce strain on the joints in the low back.

Reclining in a supported position

When sitting reclined, try to support your back to help the low back maintain approximately the same shape as when standing. Lack of support will cause the low back to curve outwards while too much support using too many cushions will compress it inwards. Neither of these shapes are natural for your back and put the lumbar spine into a strained position. A reclining chair offers ideal support. Alternatively use a reclining garden chair or simply support your back in the reclined position with cushions or pillows.

Reclining chair – benefits

Patients with long-standing back pain have benefited from using a reclining chair. Being able to rest their back at the end of the day reclined, instead of sitting upright, has significantly improved their condition. When deciding on recliners I advise trying them out before buying. The ideal recliner will support your back while maintaining the natural curve of your low back as closely as possible. Various companies make reclining chairs to accommodate people of all sizes.

Using a footstool (or putting your feet up)

Many recliner chairs have foot stools or sections that elevate the legs when the chair is in a reclined position. Similarly, if you are reclined on a sofa you will probably have your legs up. When your legs are elevated avoid having the legs straight or the muscles at the back of the legs will be pulled into tension. Any tension in the leg muscles will be transmitted through the soft tissue and into the low back and can aggravate back pain. Therefore when resting with your legs elevated, bend your knees enough to release any tension at the back of the legs.

Lying down – finding the best position

For people with back pain or neck pain lying down is normally beneficial as it removes strain from the joints in the back and neck. Release from strain means the joints, muscles and ligaments of the spine have greater opportunity to recover from an injury, or from the wear and tear of daily use.

The most frequently asked question is, "Which is the best position to use when lying down?" Most people sleep either on their side or back both of which are fine. However, a small percentage of people sleep on their front which is inadvisable for the following reasons. Lying on your front causes the abdomen to drop forward, increasing the curve in the low back. Increasing the curve in the low back puts the joints out of their relaxed position and under some strain. This causes the joints to do some work and prevents them focusing on healing and repairing themselves.

Avoid lying with the neck turned to one side

A further problem with lying on your front is that inevitably the neck will be turned to one side. When the head is turned to one side the joints in the neck are in a rotated position. This sleeping position maintained over a period of time can cause disturbance to the joints, and because the joints are not fully relaxed when the neck is held rotated, they are not properly rested.

Case Study – how your sleeping position can affect back pain

I treated a patient who worked in the building industry. For many years he had suffered with an episode of low back pain which occurred at least once a year. Over the course of many episodes he was treated by a number of different practitioners. Although these treatments helped his back pain to recover the problem reoccurred.

During an initial consultation the patient described a tendency to sleep on his front. As explained this prevents the lower back from being fully relaxed. The physical demands of his job as a builder meant it was essential to rest his back in the best position to allow it to recover from the stresses and strains that his occupation entailed. My recommendation to change his sleeping position significantly reduced the reoccurrence rate of his back pain. Four years later he needed treatment for a different complaint but confirmed that since no longer sleeping on his front he had not experienced a single episode of low back pain.

Preventing back or neck pain

Even if you do not suffer from back or neck pain I recommend that you avoid sleeping on your front as a preventative measure. For some people changing their sleeping position presents a problem due to the initial discomfort a change causes. Each time you find yourself lying on your front I suggest changing to a different position. Doing this will help change the habit of lying in that position, and you will become accustomed to a different sleeping position.

Bending and lifting – what to avoid

Most people assume they know how to bend and lift and many have had work related training. Advice on lifting tends to place the emphasis on keeping your posture upright and bending from the knees. However, there is a lack of scientific evidence in support of this approach to lifting. For instance, when a young child bends to pick an object off the ground we notice that the technique incorporates more focus on the hip joint. While bending down young children do not keep the upper body vertical, they allow the upper body to bend forward from the hip and keep the back very straight.

Avoiding overstressing the knees

If you keep your body very upright while bending, although the joints of the back are kept in line with gravity giving them some protection from the stresses of lifting, it is done at the expense of over stressing the knees. The knee is not as strong as the hip which is the strongest joint in the body and is the one most capable of absorbing the loads of bending.

Focusing all the stress of lifting in the knees over stresses them. This causes all the muscles in the leg to tense up and this tension then extends upward into the low back. If you have a sensitive back due to an injury, straining the knees will cause it to tense and should be avoided.

Case Study – overstressing the knees

A patient with an injured back came to the surgery. She was in her late thirties. The injury occurred three days earlier during a badminton match. As a mother of three young children she frequently bent down to pick things off the floor. Since the injury she bent carefully from the knees while remaining upright and keeping her back straight. This she believed was the correct way to bend. However, despite having no underlying knee problems and after using this bending method for only 3 days, she suffered from pain in both knees as well as her back pain. Despite being relatively young she had overstressed her knees through incorrect bending.

Bending from the knees becomes more difficult with age

Older people or those with any underlying knee complaint will find it even more difficult to attempt to bend using only the knees. During the bending action people with sensitive knees come to a point when it is not possible to go any lower due to discomfort and strain on the knees. At this point they will usually stoop over, bending at the waist. Bending at the waist puts a lot of strain on the low back joints and removes any benefit from bending with the knees. The result is stress on both the back and knees.
Although it is good to keep the back straight when you bend, holding the upper body upright while using only your knees is not beneficial and should be avoided.

How to achieve natural bending

The following movement will help achieve a natural bending action. When you want to pick something up imagine there is a chair behind you which you are going to sit on. Sitting in a chair is completed in two actions, firstly we bend forward at the hip, and slightly flex out the knees, so that our upper body is at an angle inclining forward, secondly we bend further at the knee to lower ourselves into the chair. When standing the body should naturally bend forward from the hip to bend, in exactly the same as the first action of sitting. As long as you avoid looking down too much or dropping your chest, and imagine you are doing the first part of the sitting action, you will find you naturally bend forward from the hip and keep your back straight.

Picking something up correctly

To pick something off the floor simply extend the movement until you touch the floor. As you bend down if your knees come in front of the toes then you are not letting yourself bend from the hips enough and are over stressing your knees. Regaining the correct movement can take a little practice, but because it is a natural action the more you do it the more automatic it becomes.

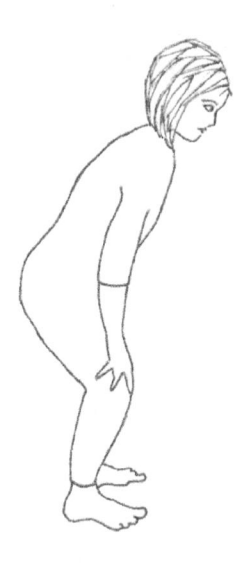

Maintaining hip mobility

Keeping the hips flexible is vital to enable the body to bend correctly. I have included some useful exercises in chapter 12 to help maintain hip mobility.

Chapter 8
Pain in the middle and upper back

Restriction and lack of mobility cause pain in the middle and upper back

The area of the back immediately above the inward curve of the low back upwards to the base of the neck is known as the thoracic spine, or more commonly the middle and upper back. The bones (vertebra) that form the spine in the middle and upper back support and anchor the rib cage. The attachment of the ribs to this area of the spine has the effect of profoundly restricting the movement of the middle and upper back. The limited nature of natural movement in the middle and upper back cause this area to be prone to problems associated with tension and loss of flexibility.

Stiffness in the middle and upper back – can cause acute strain and pain

This tendency for the mid and upper back to be very stiff can cause two common problems.

Firstly, lack of suppleness and give in the joints can predispose them to acute strains.

Secondly, if restriction and tightness builds up too much it can cause pain even without an injury. Chronic tension can cause compaction and pressure within the joints causing pain. In addition muscles, ligaments and tendons are not meant to sustain high levels of tension indefinitely and will become irritable and inflamed if they become chronically tense.
Problems in the middle and upper back related to tension and stiffness do not normally cause permanent damage. As long as the problem is treated before it has become too chronic it is generally easy to resolve. A program of exercises that selectively loosen the areas of tightness can be effective.

However, when areas of the middle and upper back have become very restricted, the individual will require help from professionals such a chiropractor, physiotherapist or osteopath who can apply techniques that loosen and release areas of restriction and tension.

Developing a strong, relaxed breathing pattern – good for loosening the middle/upper back and preventing tightness in the chest

Developing a strong, relaxed breathing pattern ensures good movement of the ribcage during breathing. This helps keep the middle back, upper back and rib cage relaxed and loose.
How to achieve this is explained on page 141 in Chapter 10

Loosening exercises - good for the middle and upper back

To loosen your middle and upper back, I recommend trying each of the following exercises and then selecting the three or four exercises that seem to be the most helpful.

Please note: during the first few days of an injury there may be significant inflammation, therefore loosening and stretching exercises should be carried out as gentle movements. That is gently and slowly moving into and out of the exercise positions, without pushing into a stretch. This will loosen the area while avoiding irritation. As mentioned above if the tense area is long-standing it may be too tight to release through exercise alone and may need professional help.

Exercise 1

Arm Brushing – good for loosening the shoulders and upper back and a warm up for other exercises

To start hold the arms fairly straight and palms loosely together in front of you.

Now move one palm up the inside of the other arm into the shoulder, over the shoulder and down the outside of the arm to the back of the hand, then back over the finger tips onto the palms. This brings you back to the start position (As you come down the back of the arm it helps to slightly curve your fingers to lightly cup the back of the arm).

Without stopping continue the movement a number of times, and then repeat on the other arm.

There should be some gentle rotation of the body and swinging of the arm as you do this exercise. Try to relax and let your body move naturally.

As you move upwards on the inside of the arm, the arm should swing backward. As you progress down the outside of the arm the arm should swing forward again.

When brushing your hand over the body, aim for a feeling similar to rubbing your hands together to create static electricity. Try to use one continuous movement, relax and try to avoid rushing.

Pain in the middle and upper back

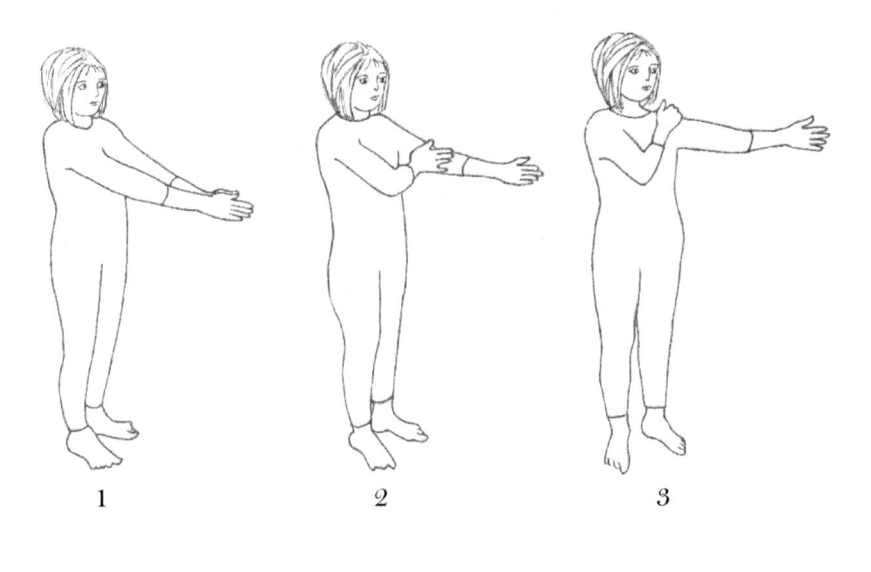

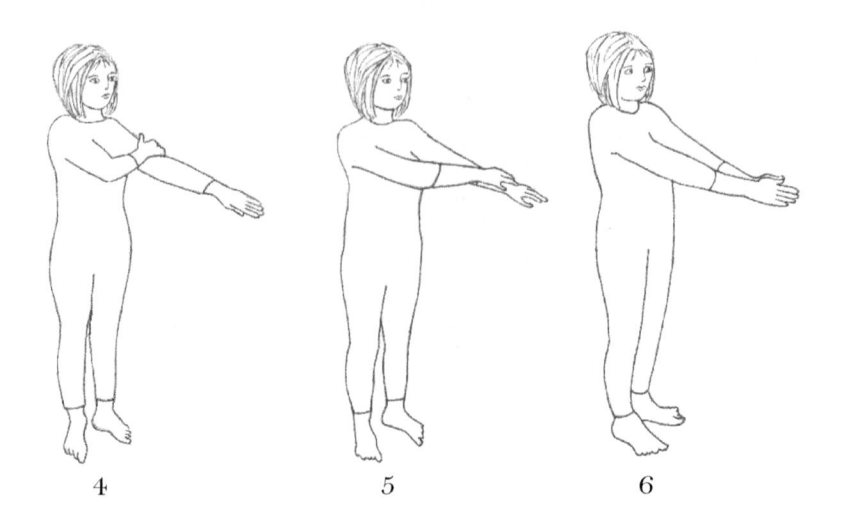

1

2

3

4

5

6

Exercises that cause lifting of the rib cage

Good for loosening the ribcage and shoulders

Good for improving mobility in the whole back

The ribs form a protective cage around the internal organs in the upper body, but in performing this function the ribs restrict movement of the spine. Exercises which cause the rib cage to stretch upward stretch the soft tissues holding the ribs in place and improve the back's mobility.

Exercises to release shoulder and neck tension

In the section on posture (Chapter 10) I identify a key problem with posture which is the tendency for people to slump forward with the upper body. As a result the ribs become compressed and tight, pulling forward the neck and shoulders, leading to shoulder and neck tension.

The following two exercises involve lifting the rib cage and are good for regaining the sense of stretch and length in the upper body. This helps release any pull on the neck and shoulders allowing them to assume their correct position.

Exercise 2

Arm Swing – good for loosening the back, shoulders and ribcage

To start adopt a standing position letting both arms swing forward and back at the side of the body.

To keep the arms and shoulders as relaxed as possible try to maintain the movement by gently stretching the fingers as the arms swing in front of the body.

Relax the arms and hands as they reach the top of the swing at the front. From the top of the swing in front of the body, totally relax the arms and hands so they naturally swing down and back behind you.

As the arms swing forward from behind, repeat again gently stretching the fingers as the hands come in front of you. Try to catch the timing of the swing so that you put the effort in at the right point to build the swing up without interrupting the movement.

Try to gently increase the swing in this way so the arms rise above your head at the front.

Continue this exercise for several minutes. Stop if it becomes uncomfortable.

You will feel that the movement of the arms causes the rib cage to rise and fall. This lifting and falling movement of the rib cage loosens the tissues around the ribs and back.

You can bring your whole body into this exercise by relaxing your hips as you let the arms swing down and back, then straightening the hips to help swing the arms up and forward again.

Pain in the middle and upper back

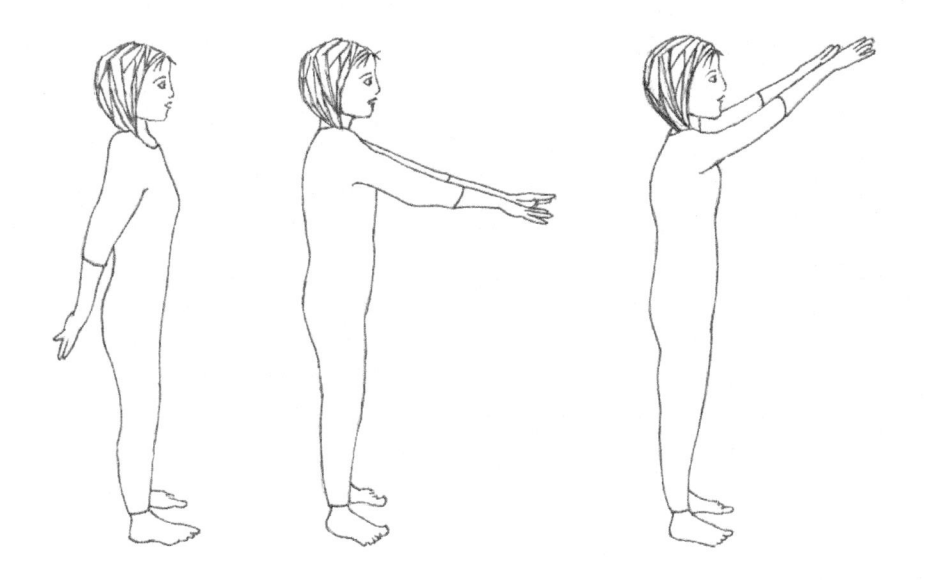

Exercise 3

Stretching the arms above the head – good for creating stretch in the rib cage

To start stretch your arms vertically upwards over your head so they are parallel.

Bend your wrists back and turn your hands so the fingers are pointing toward each other with the little fingers at the back.

Stretch the hands and fingers, bending the wrists back as you reach up encourages more lift in the rib cage.

Hold at the top for about 5 seconds. If you hold too long it can cause the shoulders to tense up.

After about 5 seconds stretching up in this position relax your arms down so your hands are level with the top of your head.

After a short pause repeat the exercise.
You can do this exercise in sets of 5 to 10 repetitions.

Additional similar exercise – good for loosening the rib cage

To start stretch one arm up whilst stretching the opposite arm vertically down.

Bend the wrists back with the fingers of each hand pointing towards each other but this time on the hand stretching down the little finger is at the front.

The arm stretching down holds that side of the ribs down, whilst the opposite hand stretching up lifts its side of the rib cage up.

Hold for about 5 seconds, repeat 5 to 10 times on each side

This creates a useful stretch between each side of the rib cage.

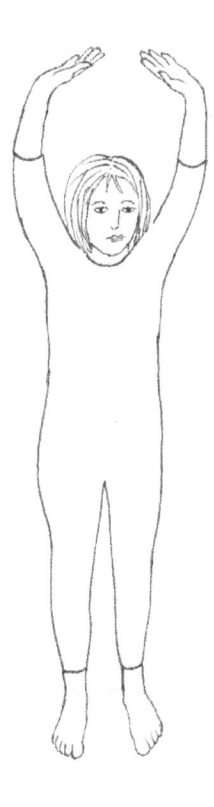

Pain in the middle and upper back

Exercise 4

Sitting twist – good for stretching the upper body

When you twist the body in the standing position most of the rotation occurs at the waist and lower body. To stretch the upper body in a twist the exercise is best done sitting down. Sitting restricts the movement of the waist and lower body so that any stretch is more focused around the rib cage and mid/upper back area.

Once your arms are in the required position, remember to relax your arms and shoulders before commencing the twist.

Twist to stretch the upper back

If you twist with your elbows bent facing upwards and your fingertips touching behind your neck, the focus of the twist will be more at the top of your back.

Twist to stretch the middle of the back

If you place each hand on the opposite shoulder so the arms are crossed in front of you and twist, the stretch is focused more in the middle of the back.

Twist to stretch the lower mid back

If you move the arms down to waist level and place each hand on the opposite elbow and twist while seated in this position, you will find the focus of the stretch is lower again around the bottom of the rib cage.

You can stretch the whole mid and upper back by doing these three stretches as a series.

Hold each stretch for 3 or 4 breaths and repeat each one 3 or 4 times to each side.

Pain in the middle and upper back

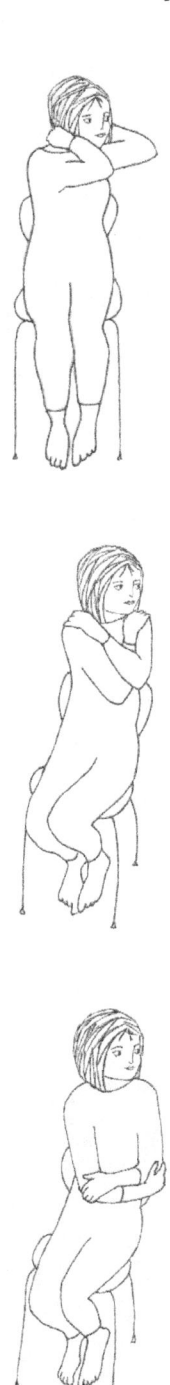

Exercise 5

Stretching to the side – good for increasing mobility in the whole of the back

When the rib cage becomes tight and restricted, stretching to the side is a good way to open up and loosen the side of the rib cage and increase mobility in the whole back.

Stretching to the side can be done seated, but for most people it is easier from the standing position.

To start stand with 90% of your weight on one leg. This has the effect of stiffening the waist so that when you stretch to the side the stretch is focused in the rib cage and upper body, and not in the waist.

From the starting position, with 90% of your weight on one leg, stretch the arm on the side where the weight is, over your head to the opposite side, while maintaining 90% weight on the leg.

Keep the opposite leg straight or your body will tend to twist.
You should feel the rib cage opening up and stretching.

If you wish you can slightly change the focus of the stretch by having the palm of your hand either pointing towards the floor or to the ceiling during the stretch. You may find one of the two hand positions gives a more positive stretch to your tight areas.

When you achieve a comfortable stretch relax in the position and take a few deep slow breaths, which will help to loosen the rib cage further.

Try holding the stretch for 3 or 4 breaths and repeat 3 or 4 times to each side.

Pain in the middle and upper back

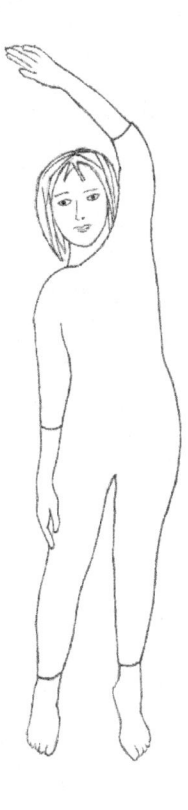

Exercise 6

Stretching arms out to the side – good for loosening around the shoulders

To start stretch the arms out to each side so they are slightly raised to about fifteen degrees above your shoulders. This slight upward angle improves the stretch in the shoulders.

Bend the wrists back towards ninety degrees and stretch the fingers. This action also improves the effectiveness of the exercise.

Hold for a few seconds, then relax the hands and arms but without letting them drop very far.

As you relax the arms imagine you are trying to grip a pencil between your shoulder blades. The act of contracting your shoulder blades together stimulates the muscles there. This causes a relaxation of the trapezius muscles on the top of the shoulders through a reflex action.

After squeezing the shoulder blades together in this way for a few seconds, go back to the first part of the exercise, stretching the arms out again.

These movements can be repeated 5 to 10 times as is comfortable. It is very effective in loosening the area around the shoulders.

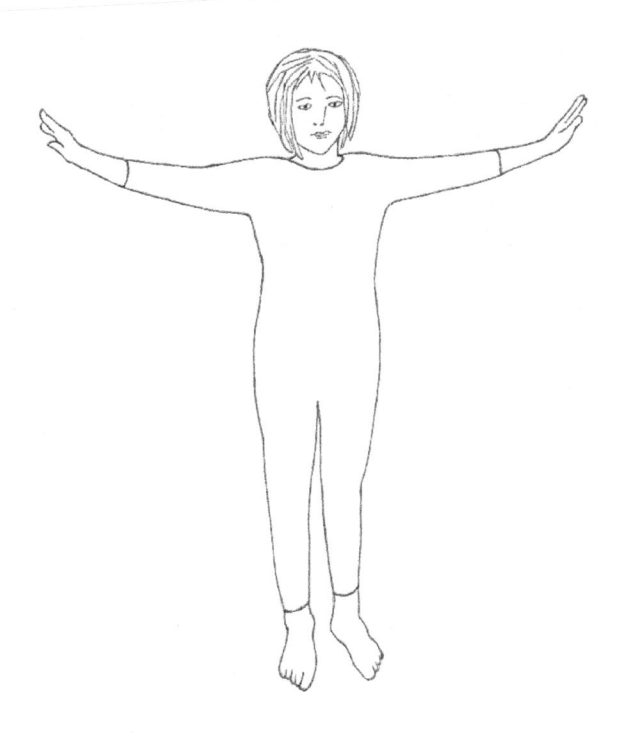

Pain in the middle and upper back

Pain to one side of the spine and/or radiating around the rib cage

This type of pain is often caused by disturbance of the rib cage. As with upper back pain, pain from the ribs is most frequently due to either a build up of tension and restriction, or some incident causing a strain.

Disturbance to the ribs can be felt as pain at any point along the ribs, from their starting point to one side of the spine, to where they attach to the sternum in the middle of the chest.

What to do
Exercises for strains to the rib cage

You can slightly adapt the exercises used for releasing tightness in the mid and upper back. These exercises are, swinging the arms, stretching over head, sitting twist and stretching to the side, all of which are described earlier in this chapter.

Adapting the sitting twist and side stretch exercises for treating a rib strain

Slightly adjust the sitting twist and side stretch exercises by doing them towards the good side only.
These exercises are done towards the good side only because in some cases of rib cage disturbance, doing a stretch on the opposite side from the injury towards the painful side causes compression of the injured area which sometimes aggravates the problem.

Therefore, start by doing the sitting twist and side stretch towards the good side only. If your pain is on the right you do the twist and side stretch to the left only, which will stretch and open up the injured area.

Do the stretches gently and if there is no negative reaction you can also do them towards the painful side to see if this helps.
If there is a negative reaction go back to doing the exercises towards the pain free side only.

Pain between or around the shoulder blades

Pain felt between or just inside the shoulder blade, or on top of the shoulder is another common problem that manifests in the upper back. This can be a localised problem in the joints or muscles of the upper back but is frequently caused by a problem in the neck.

Signs that pain in the upper back are originating from the neck

There can be many indications that pain in the upper back is coming from the neck rather than where the pain is being felt. Firstly when there is also pain in the shoulder, arm or hand. Another sign is when you try to stretch the painful area to release tension, it either makes no difference or seems to aggravate the problem.

Patients tend to describe it as "I've got this really tight muscle behind my shoulder blade. My partner tried some massage on it but it does not make any difference. I was hoping you could apply some stronger massage". Or they may have had professional massage treatment to the upper back which either made no difference, or aggravated the symptoms. When any of these signs are present I usually find an examination of the patient's neck will reveal a possible cause.

For treatment go to Chapter 9, Relieving neck pain

If this sounds familiar and trying various exercises and treatments has not resolved pain in your upper back or shoulders, go to the end of chapter 9 for advice on treating these types of symptoms.

Pain in the middle and upper back

Chapter 9
Relieving Neck pain

Avoid looking down

A neck injury will be aggravated by any activity that involves looking down. Looking down causes the neck to flex forward, putting a strain on the neck joints and will aggravate most types of neck injury. Activities such as reading, writing, housework and many creative pursuits for instance, sewing or painting require you to look down.

As the head tilts forward to look down it is no longer over the middle of the neck. When the head is no longer cantered over the neck it is no longer in a stable position and naturally falls forward. This puts a strain on the neck joints and causes the muscles at the back of the neck to tense up to hold the head in position.

Acute neck pain

Treatment Options: manual therapy, medication, a cold pack

In the first few days the best approach is to let the injury settle naturally. If the condition is excessively painful there are techniques a manual therapist such as a chiropractor, physiotherapist or osteopath can use to help reduce the pain, or medication can be obtained from your family doctor.

Self Help

For the first few days of the injury it is usually better to use a cold pack on the area rather than heat, see the end this Chapter for further details.

It is also vital to protect the injury from unnecessary stress. Avoid any activity where you are holding the neck in a strained position. For example, flexing the neck forward (looking down), backward (looking up) or twisting (looking to one side).

Neck injury and the "guarding" effect

The neck normally has good natural mobility due to the way the head follows the movement of the eyes. Each time you look at something the head and neck will turn in that direction. This constant movement of the neck normally maintains a good level of flexibility in the neck joints.

However, if one of the joints in the neck is injured the muscles around the neck will tighten causing the neck to feel stiff, a process called guarding.

Guarding is when the body itself causes contraction and tightening around an injured area of the body. The function of guarding is to restrict movement and stress on a damaged joint or area of the body.

In most cases of neck injury where the muscles of the neck have become tense, there is nothing wrong with the muscles, they are simply trying to protect some deeper injury. If you try and stretch them or force movement in the early stages of an injury, you are going against the body's natural healing mechanism which will often aggravate the situation.

Orthopaedic collar - good for limiting stress on a neck injury

If you have a neck injury, dropping the head forward causes pain and slows recovery. During an activity involving looking down it is easy to forget not to drop your head forward. Wearing an orthopaedic collar during these types of activities prevents the head dropping forward too much and limits the stress on a neck injury. Made from soft foam orthopaedic collars are light, yet firm enough to limit how far you can tilt your head forward

For most types of common neck injury a shallow collar is ideal because it does not stop you moving your head entirely and the collar serves to limit movement if you try to look down, preventing the head tilting forward too much. Collars are available from pharmacists and orthopaedic suppliers.

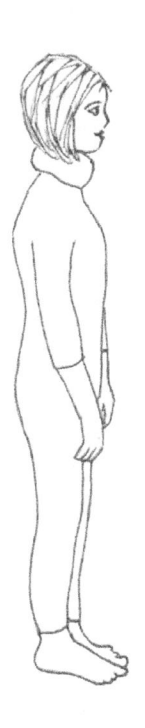

Should I exercise my neck when I have acute pain?

In the early stages of a neck injury, trying to force the neck will cause irritation. Professional therapists such as chiropractors, osteopaths and physiotherapists are able to treat the area around the injury without irritating it.

For people trying to manage the problem themselves it is best to be cautious. In my experience the head lift is one of the few exercises that may usually be used safely by people with a very sensitive neck injury. The head lift gently separates the joints in the neck, releasing pressure and tension. Please see the next page for details.

Exercise

Head lift - good for most types of neck pain

A simple but effective exercise for acute or chronic neck pain and also for pain referred from the neck into the arm, shoulder, or upper back.

To start adopt the standing position.
Place one hand on each side of the head with the heel of your hands slightly hooked under the angle of the jaws. Try to lift your head straight upwards and avoid pushing it backward. This action should be done quite gently yet firmly enough to feel a stretch in the neck muscles.

Hold for 3 to 5 seconds then relax, repeat 3 to 5 times.

If you find the exercise helpful you can do it several times through the day but leave at least two hours between each set.

If this exercise seems to aggravate your condition do not continue.

Please note neck injuries can be easily aggravated by unsuitable exercises but most acute neck injuries will settle naturally as long as they are not subject to too much strain. Therefore if you have an acute neck injury I would advise a professional assessment before trying other neck exercises.

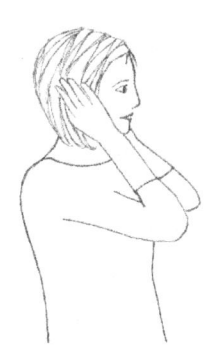

Chronic long term neck pain

Chronic neck pain can be very difficult to treat because the neck is in constant motion. Your head moves continuously to follow your gaze which in turn generates continuous movement and stress to the neck. If your neck suffers significant injury, the constant strain to damaged tissue, caused by the neck's natural movements, can slow or impair healing.

Improving posture
Good for encouraging healing, reducing neck pain.

To encourage healing, you need to protect your injured neck from unnecessary strain. The most effective means of protecting your neck is through correct posture. For instance, when watching television sitting on the couch or armchair we tend to drop the head forward, causing strain on the neck. Similarly computer screens are often too low so the head is tilted forward, again placing unnecessary strain on the neck. We place these kinds of unnecessary stresses on our neck without even realising. When the neck is suffering from a long term injury the correct posture can be essential to recovery.

See Chapter 7 for advice on how to set up your desk correctly.

When relaxing at home you should ensure your neck is fully supported as explained in Chapter 10. This chapter explains the importance of posture to recovery.

Headaches and dizziness

Studies suggest 80% of headaches are caused by tension or disturbances in the neck. Dizziness is also a frequent side effect of disturbance to the neck.

If you suffer from headaches or dizziness and other causes have been eliminated, it is advisable to consult a chiropractor, osteopath or physiotherapist.

Exercises for reducing neck stiffness

Stiffness in the neck without the experience of significant pain is more usual in older people. With age the joints tend to gradually tighten causing stiffness. If you feel you cannot move your neck as much as you would like, and do not have significant pain, some of the exercises on the next few pages may help.

Avoid overworking injured tissues

If you have a neck injury rather than age related stiffness, general neck exercises such as those included here should be avoided as they can exacerbate the problem.

The constant natural movement and stress involved in daily living is usually enough strain for any neck injury to cope with.

Avoid general non-specific exercise, which can overwork injured tissues and interfere with healing. It is advisable to consult a professional such as a chiropractor, osteopath or physiotherapist for exercises specifically for your condition.

Starting gently

Because age related neck stiffness can be sensitive to exercise, I recommend starting with short exercise sessions, varying the amount according to how your neck reacts.

Focus on the exercises you feel comfortable with, moving on to more challenging exercises if your neck feels receptive.

The neck can be particularly sensitive to exercise and should you have any problems it is advisable to seek professional advice.

Exercise

Head lean to the side – good for neck stiffness

To start lean your body slightly to one side, then lean your head to that same side and relax it. Lean your head as far as is comfortable.

You should feel a stretch down the opposite side of the neck.

You can increase the stretch further by leaning more to the side or by bringing your arm up on the side you are leaning towards and placing your hand on your head. Don't pull your head down, keep your arm relaxed and let the extra weight of your arm and hand provide extra stretch.

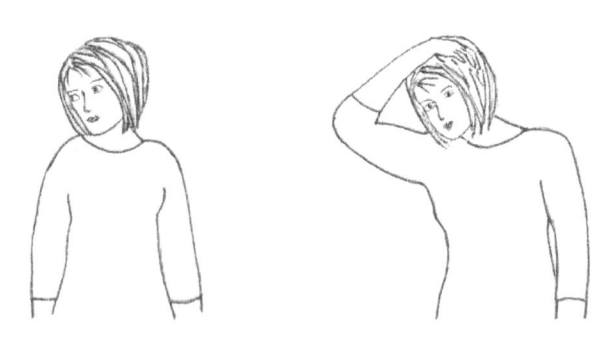

Head lean to one corner - good for neck stiffness

To start let the head lean over at an angle, half way between leaning it over to the side as before and dropping forward.

As before you can use the weight of the arm to increase the stretch, but this time lift the arm up from the direction you are stretching towards when placing the hand on the head.

For either of the neck lean exercises do up to 4 repetitions to each side, holding each for about 3 breaths.

If your neck is sensitive reduce the amount of repetitions.

Exercise

Forward semicircle neck roll – good for a stiff neck

A normal neck roll, in which you roll the head round in a complete circle, can be too aggressive for someone with a stiff neck. The following is an easier variation of the exercise.

It can be done sitting or standing but my patients find it easier standing.

To start let your head relax forward and allow it to hang there relaxed.

Keeping your head and neck completely relaxed, roll your head slowly to the left. When you reach about 45 degrees you will feel how the movement becomes more difficult and more force is needed to continue. Stop at this point and slowly roll the head back down through the central point again.

Continue to the other side until you reach the point at about 45 degrees where the movement becomes difficult. Stop at this point and roll the head back down and to the first side again.

Do 6 to 8 repetitions to each side or less if they start to become uncomfortable.

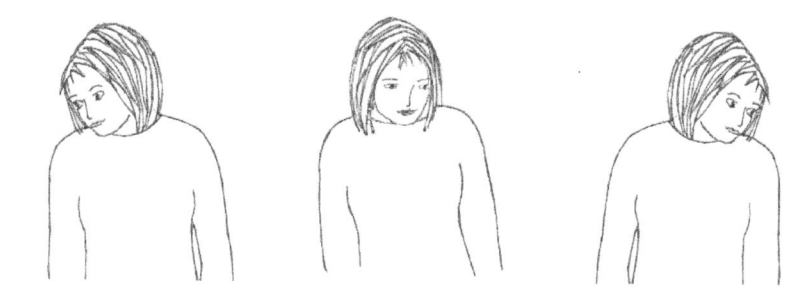

Exercise

Looking to each side – good for a stiff neck

To twist the head to each side, begin by looking to one side with your eyes instead of actually twisting your neck. The head will automatically turn in that direction and follow your gaze, in a natural relaxed way.

If you try and obtain the same movement by focusing on twisting the neck to the side although you end up with the same movement, it can create more tension in the neck muscles.

Do up to 5 repetitions to each side, holding for 2 or 3 breaths.

Pain in the arm, hand, shoulder or between the shoulder blades caused by a neck injury

Referred pain – what is it?

When you have an injured joint in the neck it can often cause nerve irritation leading to symptoms in the arm, hand, shoulder or between the shoulder blades. This is because the nerve supply to these areas stems from the lower part of the neck. When an injury in the neck causes pain elsewhere it is known as referred pain. For referred pain to occur the neck does not always have to feel particularly painful.

Because the neck may not feel the most painful area, referred pain from the neck can easily be interpreted as a shoulder problem or a pulled muscle in the back.

Signs of referred pain

If pain in the arm, hand, shoulder or between the shoulder blades is coming from the neck, you will know it is referred pain if you experience the following:

1. The nerves in the neck come out of the side of the neck joints. Gently feel down the side of your neck for sensitive areas, particularly at the bottom of the neck where the neck meets the top of the shoulder. Any sensitivity should relate to the side of the body where the symptoms are being felt.

2. Pain symptoms in the upper back which are not eased by massage or stretching or are aggravated by these activities, are often a sign that the pain is being referred from the neck. Usually tense muscles or joints in the upper back can be eased by stretching or massage.

3. If you have pain in the shoulder due to a shoulder injury there will be significant stiffness and loss of movement. If you have shoulder pain but without any significant stiffness or loss of movement, the pain is most likely to be due to referred pain from another area, probably the neck.

These are some of the signs of referred pain which can indicate that pain felt in the arm, hand, shoulder or between the shoulder blades is coming from nerve irritation in the neck.

How to treat pain referred from the neck

When you have a neck injury that is causing pain in other areas of the body, it normally means the injury is very sensitive and easily aggravated. Although you may not have much pain in the neck it should be treated in the same way as acute neck pain, described at the beginning of this chapter.

In brief, avoid positions of stress in the neck (looking up, down or to the side)
Use a soft collar to protect your neck from tilting forward during activities involving looking down.

Try the head lift exercise described earlier in this chapter.

Applying an ice pack to the neck – good for acute neck pain and pain referred from the neck

If you find the side of the neck is very sensitive, applying an ice pack to this area often helps (ice packs are widely available from pharmacists, alternatively use a bag of frozen peas).

To use an ice pack place a thin layer of material over the ice pack, such as a T shirt and apply to the side of the neck making sure you include the lower part of the neck where it meets the shoulder. This is easiest to do whilst lying on the opposite side, as the ice pack will stay in position without being held.

Apply the ice pack for short periods of about 5 minutes at a time, and no more than once an hour. Over chilling the neck may cause it to tense up and reduce the beneficial effect.
Further information on use of ice packs is given at the end of Chapter 12

Chapter 10
Posture

The stresses and strains we experience as a result of living in the twenty first century can lead us to develop posture that is unbeneficial. It is never too late however, to correct posture and invest in gradual improvements which can significantly improve back and neck pain, and increase well being and energy levels. Moreover, these improvements can easily be included in the working day which benefits people whose work prevents them allocating time to specific exercises.

The benefits of good posture

Reduces strain on joints which can have a beneficial effect on injuries, such as those causing back or neck pain.

Reducing strain on joints also helps prevent long term wear and tear which reduces the risk of arthritis.

Poor posture wastes energy. Good posture is efficient because it entails less effort which increases energy levels and enables you to do more before you get tired.

Improving posture will help you use your body more effectively, making you less likely to injure your back or neck during activities.

Good posture reduces neck and back pain

For people with worn or chronically injured joints developing good posture is an essential means of reducing pain. When for example, we fracture a bone, or severely tear a ligament or tendons, the area is put in a cast. This support assists tissue repair by reducing the stresses on the injury. Similarly, good posture minimises strain on joints and assists the healing process.

Good posture reduces stress on an injury and assists recovery

During a normal day, reducing the overall stress put on an injury will significantly assist recovery and can be achieved through minor adjustments to your posture. With a long-standing problem any minor adjustments to posture may seem too subtle to make a difference. Studies show however that improvements to posture, particularly in the workplace, can have a major impact on chronic back or neck pain.

Adjusting posture in the hips

Stretching and relaxing the hips – good for relaxing the posture

Why?

Tension around the hip joints is a common problem causing incorrect posture. We know for instance, that in young children their bending movement is centred round the hip joint but as we grow older we tend to become stiff around the hips. As a result when we move or bend our hips are restricted so that more of the movement has to occur in the low back. My experience treating patients indicates that restriction in the hips is one of the main causes of low back injuries.

Stiffness in the hips transfers the stress of movement and bending from the hips to the low back. Correcting this condition by loosening the hip joints means bending and moving will occur naturally again at the hip joint, thereby protecting the low back from over use. Releasing tension and regaining flexibility in the hip joints can also have other profound effects on posture. All the main muscle groups in the lower body and back are attached to or are affected by the hips, causing tension in the hips to be transferred through the whole body. It follows that releasing hip tension will reduce tension throughout the body.

Tension in the hips also pulls the posture off balance, most commonly it causes a shift in weight from the centre of the feet toward the heels. If you rock back on your heels you may feel how this increases tension in the legs and low back, as well as reducing stability in the posture. Exercises that loosen the hip joints help realign posture by placing the weight over the centre of the feet.

Finally, when the hips and low back muscles are tight, the muscle tension often pulls on the low back so the natural curve is accentuated or diminished. There are various opinions on how to correct this, for instance by consciously adjusting the pelvis. However, actively adjusting the pelvic position means having to sustain unnatural levels of tension in other muscle groups to hold the corrected position. For my patients the most effective approach is loosening and relaxing the hip joints, which gradually releases excess tension in muscle groups around the pelvis and low back. Once tension is released the joints will fall back into their natural position, and any distortions caused by muscle tension will correct themselves.

How to stretch and relax the hip joints

Exercise

Simple hip release exercise – good for loosening hips and relieving low back pain.

The following gentle exercise is one I frequently use with patients to help loosen and relax the hips and is suitable for everyone.

To start stand with the inside edges of the feet approximately parallel and about 8-12 inches apart (approximately the length of one of your own feet).

Locate the hip joint in the groin by placing the palm of your right hand over your right groin area. (see next page)
Place the back of your left hand behind your back over your right buttock, directly behind the right hand but at the back of the body.

Slowly transfer more of your body weight onto your right leg. As you transfer weight onto the right side of the body more weight is transferred into the right hip. Note any sensations this transfer of

Posture

weight causes in the hip area by focusing your attention on the area between your hands.

Continue transferring the weight slowly onto the right leg in this way until you have about 80% of your weight on your right leg. Slowly transfer your weight back to the centre and again try to feel for the sensations this causes in the hip. Repeat several times then try the same exercise on the left hip.

Initially it may be difficult to feel any changes but through practising the exercise you will gradually start to develop sensitivity to the hip movement. You will feel the hip moving and notice how the movement you are practising has the effect of releasing tension in the muscles around the hip joint.

Reaching this level of sensitivity to the hip movement can be seen as a long term goal. In the meantime regular practice of the exercise has other significant benefits such as loosening the hips, relieving low back pain and ultimately reducing tension in your posture.

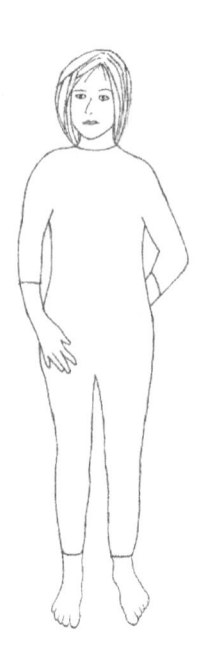

Exercise

Hip stretches, supported by a wall – good for loosening hips, pelvis and low back (see chapter 12)

The additional exercises in chapter 12, lying on the floor with the legs raised against a wall are good for stretching and loosening the hips, pelvis, and low back.

Hip stretch 1 in side position – good for stretching the hip joints

To start lie on your side on a comfortable surface.
Make sure your body is in line with one leg on top of the other.

Bend the lower leg as this helps keep the position stable. Lift the top leg straight up, keeping it in line with the body.

When you have lifted the leg as far as you can comfortably, try to stretch a little further for about 2 seconds, then lower the leg completely and relax.

It is important to relax the leg down between repetitions to keep the hip from tensing up.

Repeat up to ten times as is comfortable, one to three times a day.

Please note: When lifting the leg upwards avoid bringing the leg forward out of line with the body. The leg will go further but the stretch on the hip is not as effective.

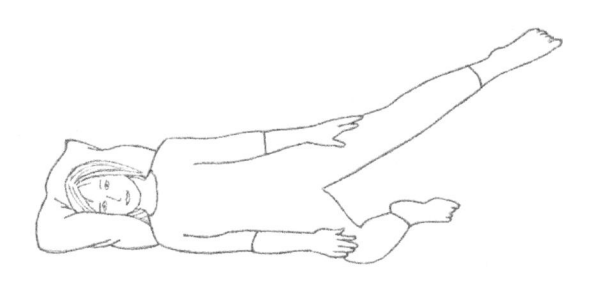

Hip stretch 2 in side position – good for stretching the hip joints

To start lie on your side as before with the lower leg bent and keeping the top leg straight, bring the top leg forward as far as you can while keeping the leg straight.

Still keeping the top leg straight, gently lower the leg to the ground and rest for a few seconds.

From holding your leg forward, bring the leg back and stretch it behind you as far as you can comfortably while keeping the leg straight. Again at the end of the movement, keeping the leg straight gently lower the leg to the ground and rest for a few seconds.

While stretching do not strain so much that your low back is pulled significantly out of shape
Repeat up to ten times as is comfortable, one to three times a day.

A pillow support

If at each end of the movement, when the leg is far forward or backward, it is uncomfortable to lower the leg, a cushion can be placed to rest the leg on as it is lowered towards the floor.

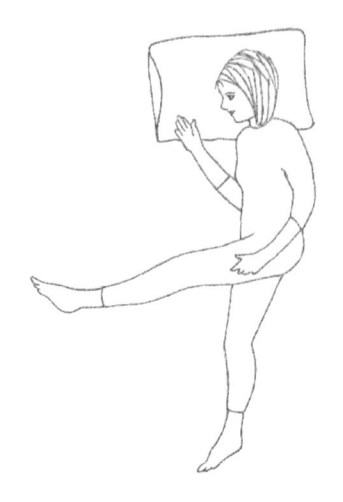

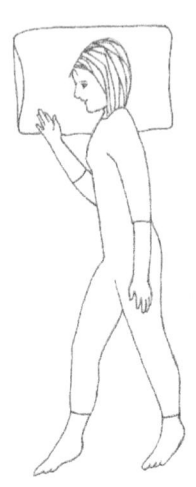

Improving the walking action - good for preventing worn knee joints, hip joints, fallen arches and tension in the low back

Foot alignment

When running or walking the weight should be placed along the middle of the foot. While walking focus your attention on the action of your feet. This will help you to feel where the weight is on the feet.

If your feet are pointing outwards as you walk you will feel the weight tending to be along the inside edge of the feet. If the feet are pointing inwards you will feel how the weight is on the outside of the feet.

Finding the correct foot position during walking

Without looking at your feet, as you walk try slightly changing your foot angle between these two positions, slightly pointing outwards and slightly pointing inwards.

Now try to find the position where you feel the weight is moving down the middle of the foot as you walk. When you have found this position your feet should be positioned with the inside edges approximately parallel.

Most people tend to walk with their feet pointing outwards too much.

At first when you correct the position with the weight over the middle of the feet, you may feel as if your feet are pointing inwards even though when you look down you can see they are not. This is because the brain is used to accepting an incorrect position as normal. Practising the correct walking position will induce the brain to adapt to the new position and accept it as normal.

Feet pointing outwards too much causes worn knee joints and tightness in the lower back.

When the feet are pointing outwards too much, weight is transferred down the inside of the leg causing the inside part of the knee joint to become worn.

The resulting wear on the knee joint can make an early knee replacement necessary. There is also increased weight over the arch of the foot which can cause problems.

Another problem caused by the feet pointing outwards is rotation of the hip joint, leading to shortening in the ligaments across the back of the pelvis and subsequent tightness in the low back.

Correct positioning of the feet reduces wear on the knee joints and tension in the back

When the feet are in the correct position with the inside edges roughly parallel, the weight is over the middle of the foot allowing the arch to lift naturally. The knee and hip joints are loaded symmetrically reducing wear. The pelvis is open at the back helping to maintain length in the pelvic ligaments that run across the low back.

Benefits of the correct stride length

Wearing shoes enables us to take longer strides, causing the foot to hit the ground with the heel first and the leg almost straight. Without shoes this would be uncomfortable. To discover this for yourself walk quickly barefoot across a tiled or concrete floor. If your stride length is too long your heels will start to feel bruised and painful.
People who walk and run without shoes naturally take shorter strides by comparison.

Benefits of the shorter stride – reduces jarring, improves balance and control

With shorter strides the foot lands on the middle and heel of the foot almost at the same time with the knee joint slightly bent. This allows the knee, ankle and foot joints to cushion and absorb the shock of landing much more efficiently than when the leg is straight. It is a much softer way of moving and there is less jarring at the moment the foot strikes the ground.

Walking or running without an overly long stride also gives the body a greater sense of control, allowing your whole posture to feel more relaxed. You can experience this by experimenting with walking and changing the length of your strides from short to long then back again.

Many world class athletes use a short stride in training as it has been shown to reduce injury. Well known sports brands design running shoes which reflect this approach.

How to find your correct stride length

Try taking a step extremely slowly, just an inch at a time, controlling every part of the movement. If your stride is too long you will find you cannot transfer weight slowly from one foot to the other and retain balance and control. You will be forced to make a slight leap from one foot to the other. Experiment to find the longest step you can take while being able transfer your body weight from one foot to the other, smoothly and under control, even if transferring your weight very slowly. This movement provides a guide to the approximate length of your stride. If your stride is the correct length your knees will not be locked straight when your foot lands on the ground.

Correcting upper body alignment - good for relieving shoulder and neck tension

Avoid slumping forward

The collapsing down of the rib cage is possibly the most common problem with the upper body posture. Most people tend to slump forward so their rib cage is collapsed at the front, pulling the shoulders and head forward.

To rectify the problem people tend to stretch their neck up more or push their shoulders back. Both strategies engage other muscles and involve extra effort, creating unnecessary tension without solving the problem.

Lengthening the rib cage

Try instead to gently lift up through the ribcage and trunk without tensing. When the upper body is lengthened the ribcage is not squashed down and the shoulders and head naturally return to their correct position.

Unstable posture causes muscle tension

When standing or sitting the body should be positioned so that the skeleton is supporting our body weight. If you are slumped forward your weight and centre of gravity are no longer aligned with the skeleton, so that your posture is unstable. To compensate you will be forced to use muscle tension to hold your position.

Envisage a pole that is leaning to one side and held in position by ropes attached to it. Without the tension in the ropes the pole would fall over. Similarly we come to depend on tension in muscles to hold our posture if we are leaning out of alignment. Most people have a degree of imbalance within their posture which is held unconsciously with muscle tension.

Exercise

For realigning the posture - good for upper body and neck tension

During treatment of my patients I am constantly bending forward which pulls my posture forward out of alignment. I use this corrective exercise frequently during the day to realign my posture.

To start (fig 1) shows incorrect posture. Lift and straighten your upper body, then move your upper body (usually backwards) so it is directly over your lower body and your weight is over the middle of your feet (fig 2). Try this correcting process very gently as you breath out, try to avoid making your body tense.

When you have finished breathing out, let your upper body and shoulders relax and settle back down as you breathe in (fig 3).

Your shoulders should be over your hips and you will have a sense of your body being supported by its internal structures. You will find your posture becomes more relaxed (fig 3).

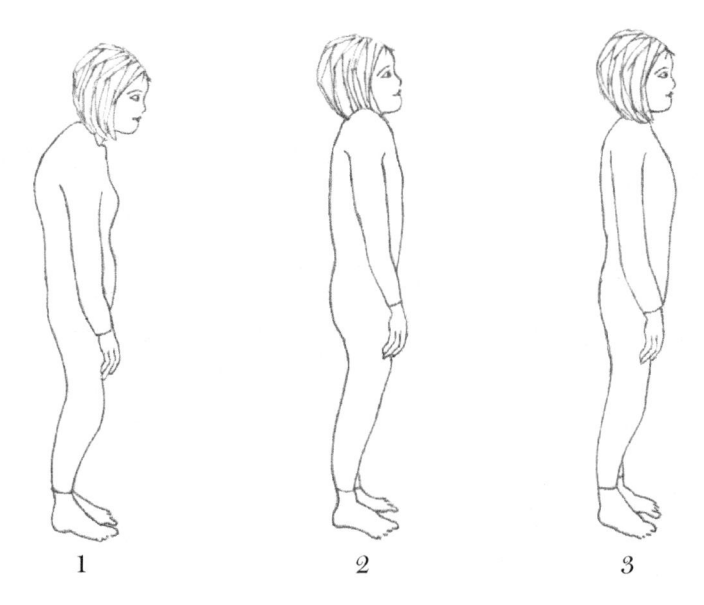

1   2   3

Exercise

An easy exercise to lengthen and lift the rib cage – good for upper body alignment

This exercise will help regain a sense of length in the ribcage and upper body.

To start stretch your arms directly upwards with the wrists bent back, approaching 90 degrees and the arms rotated so that the little fingers are facing backward and the finger tips almost touching.

In this position you should feel a strong lift and lengthening through the trunk and rib cage.
Hold for about 5 seconds then relax back down. Repeat 5-10 times

This exercise is beneficial because it produces a stretch through the upper body rarely achieved during our day to day activities.

Further exercises to loosen the upper body can be found in Chapter 8.

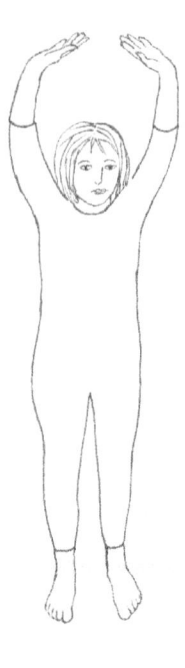

Improving neck alignment - good for relieving neck, upper back and shoulder tension.

Looking down causes tension

The majority of occupations and activities involve working with the hands which entails long periods spent looking downwards at what the hands are doing. As the head tilts forward the weight of the head moves forward until it is no longer over the neck. This is an unstable position and if not restrained the head would naturally fall forward. To stop the head dropping forward from this position the muscles in the back of the neck automatically tense. Therefore, when you look down your neck muscles are held in constant tension.

Looking down aggravates neck injuries

Holding the head forward to look down at something not only increases tension in the neck muscles it also greatly increases the stress on the neck joints. It follows that any activity which involves looking down will aggravate neck injuries.

It is advisable therefore to keep the head positioned over the middle of the neck as much as possible, with the ears roughly in line with the shoulders. This position is vital to maintaining correct neck posture.

Slumping forward stresses the neck

As mentioned previously, if you tend to let your upper body posture collapse and slump forward, this creates a pull through the muscles connecting the front of the chest to the neck and shoulders. This pulls your shoulders forward and the head forward and down, causing stress on the neck.
I recommend reading this whole chapter even if your main concern is with a problem in your neck, as incorrect posture in other areas of the body can affect the ability of the neck to be correctly positioned.

Correcting your head position

If you find you need to correct your head position, when you bring the head back over the centre of the neck, make sure you keep it level and do not end up with the chin pointing upwards. If your work involves frequent looking down, try adjusting your working position to minimise looking down while ensuring the rest of your body is comfortable.

Improving your posture at work

If you work in a sitting position, Chapter 7 explains how to set up an office chair to minimise stress on the posture. This also applies to work involving looking up or having to twist the neck to look to the side. The need to hold these positions can also result in the neck becoming overstressed.

Professional health advice – what's available

If your working position causes your neck to be held in a twist or at an angle, and improving the situation proves difficult, most major employers offer occupational health advice. Should accessing occupational health advice prove difficult, chiropractors, physiotherapists and osteopaths specialise in treating neck injuries, and have specialist knowledge of ergonomics and posture.

Relaxation - how it helps good posture

Relaxation is essential to achieving good posture. Excess muscle tension distorts the posture and unless your body is relaxed, movement cannot flow freely through the body because the joints are restricted by tension.

Daily demands can make relaxation difficult. Being in a relaxed state should not be confused with being inactive and passive which is less beneficial. You may find engaging in an enjoyable activity that releases you from your normal activities will help you to relax. There are also a wide range of self help books and CDs that can help people to relax.

In this book I have included two approaches to relaxation these are, breathing and visualisation. The information on visualisation techniques and how they assist relaxation is at the end of Chapter 5. For information on breathing as an aid to relaxation read on.

Breathing exercises - good for relaxation and good posture

Many sport and health related disciplines recognise the benefits of breathing techniques and include them in their programmes. The simple breathing techniques included here can be easily practiced at any time and will help you relax. At some stage during the day we become aware of our breathing. This awareness may occur during a quiet moment, during some kind of repetitive task, or before falling asleep at night. You can gain from these moments by using your breathing to help relax your body.

Changing the habit of shallow breathing

Whenever we become out of breath we automatically take a deep breath in. Over time this habit causes breathing in to become much stronger and more dominant than breathing out. Eventually the whole breathing cycle becomes shorter. This is because no matter how strongly you breathe in, the amount you breathe in will be limited if you have a very weak, short out breath. As a result your breathing cycle will become shallow. This is why most breathing techniques tend to focus on extending the out breath to strengthen it. This makes the breathing cycle more even and the breath slower and deeper. There are breathing techniques that suggest breathing out through the mouth to encourage the lungs to empty more completely. This can be useful as long as you don't adopt mouth breathing as a normal habit. Normal breathing should occur through the nose which has the function of warming and moistening the air before it enters the lungs.

Initially, putting more effort into breathing out might feel awkward and unnatural, but this is simply because the body has become accustomed to focussing on breathing in.

Breathing out exercise– good for extending and strengthening the out breath

Using a little extra effort make each out breath longer by one or two seconds.
This exercise needs to be done comfortably.
Avoid extending the out breath too much, or at the end of the out breath you will be left gasping for the next in breath.
Gradually extend each out breath.
This will make the in breath longer and deeper naturally.
At the end of the out breath try not to rush breathing in, relax and try to catch the natural timing of the in breath.

Breathing in exercise – good for creating a strong relaxed breathing pattern

Exercise

The urge to breathe in is both strong and natural. Therefore when you have finished breathing out try not to rush breathing in, try to catch the natural timing of the in breath. This helps stop breathing becoming too forced which can lead to hyperventilation.

Take a good full in breath but try to make the in breath slow and relaxed. When you feel the in breath has naturally finished go back to focusing on extending the out breath.

Developing a strong, relaxed breathing pattern – good for relaxation and preventing tightness in the chest and rib cage

Changing ingrained habits in the way we breathe requires regular practice in gently extending the out breath, and trying to support the in breath in a relaxed way. With practice the breathing should gradually become slower, deeper and more relaxed.

A strong relaxed breathing pattern has beneficial effects which are:
Helping to make the body more relaxed.
Regulating the correct balance of oxygen and carbon dioxide in the body.
Encouraging more movement in the rib cage preventing tightness in the chest and rib cage.

Breathing devices to strengthen breathing patterns

The "power breath"

There is help available for people who need assistance in correcting weak breathing patterns. For instance, some of my patients recommend hand held training devices, such as the "Powerbreathe." These devices are relatively inexpensive and can exercise and strengthen the muscles involved in breathing, as well as increasing lung capacity.

Question frequently asked: Can stress cause back or neck pain?

Patients frequently ask if stress is the cause of their injury. Studies reveal that stress can be a factor in a wide variety of health problems such as, heart disease, asthma, and psychological and immune related disorders. When considering back or neck pain there is little scientific evidence to support the view that stress can cause a specific, physical injury.

However, stress can increase the risk of injury. Engaging in an activity when your muscles and joints are tensed and your mind preoccupied increases the susceptibility to injury.

Similarly, if you already have an injury and are very tense due to stress, then the extra muscle tension and anxiety stress causes is likely to make your injury feel worse and have a negative effect on posture. Recent studies confirm that stress slows down the healing rate of damaged tissue, possibly due to the release of the stress hormone, cortisol and that anxiety heightens awareness of pain.

Relaxation – the key to a healthier body

The negative effect of stress on health is widely accepted and a wealth of information is available to help people cope with stress. My experience in treating patients confirms that relaxation is the key to a healthier body. Therefore I have included relaxation techniques in this chapter and at the end of Chapter 5.

Chapter 11
Healthcare Professionals – what they offer

In the treatment of back or neck pain the healthcare professionals most qualified to treat your problem are Osteopaths, Physiotherapists, Chiropractors, your family Doctor and Orthopaedic/Spinal Surgeons. Patients frequently ask how these professionals can help with their back or neck pain. To answer these questions I have summarised what they offer.

Chiropractors, Physiotherapists and Osteopaths

This group of professionals are highly qualified in diagnosis and treatment of back and neck pain. Noted for their rigorous diagnostic training and experience in the field of manual therapy they have the necessary expertise to treat many of the conditions that can lead to back and neck pain.

How to find a Chiropractor, Physiotherapist or Osteopath

Personal Recommendations
When seeking a practitioner, friends or colleagues who have been treated for back or neck pain can be a reliable source of information and able to provide a personal recommendation.

Directories
Alternatively, public information sources such as the telephone directory list practising chiropractors, physiotherapists and osteopaths. These professions are governed by legal regulations which ensure practitioners have the appropriate training and qualifications. Practitioners who advertise in a reputable directory such as the telephone directory will normally be fully qualified.

Professional registers
Chiropractors, physiotherapists and osteopaths are governed by professional bodies; these bodies have a register of qualified practitioners that can be accessed via the internet.

Treatments offered by Chiropractors, Physiotherapists and Osteopaths

These professions employ many different techniques to treat back and neck pain. My aim is to provide insight into the most commonly used approaches within chiropractic, physiotherapy and osteopathy. I will begin with diagnosis followed by methods of treatment.

Diagnosis - identifying the problem

Most back or neck pain is caused by either an accumulation of excess tension in muscles and joints, or by some form of damage to the tissues that are contained within the back or neck.
When tissues within the body are damaged through injury the tissues become inflamed and irritable which causes a protective reaction in the surrounding muscles. This muscular response is known as "guarding" and its purpose is to immobilise and protect the injured area.

The aim of treatment

If the cause of pain is some form of damage then the aim of physical treatment is to reduce the inflammation in the injured tissue and if the area around the injury has become very contracted, to try and restore normal movement. Restoring normal movement can encourage dispersal of inflammation and help to reduce excess tension.

Methods of Treatment

Ultra Sound and Mega Pulse

Electrical devices can be used to help disperse inflammation around an injury. The most common are Ultrasound and Mega Pulse.

Ultrasound uses extremely high frequency sound waves to cause agitation within the tissues. This agitation can be very effective in dispersing inflammation.

Mega-pulse uses a powerful electromagnetic field to stimulate the blood flow within the injury which can also help disperse inflammation and encourage healing.

Both Mega-pulse and Ultrasound can be useful in areas that have become sensitive and irritable. Their main advantage is that they do not cause any physical stress to the tissues under treatment and are unlikely to exacerbate a highly inflamed and sensitive injury.

Soft Tissue Work

Soft tissue work is a manual therapy which involves massaging or using pressure on the muscles, tendons or ligaments. These techniques are mostly used to reduce tension and stimulate blood flow.

Mobilisation

Among the most widely used techniques for treating back and neck pain are mobilisation and manipulation. Mobilisation is the repeated movement of any joint in the body to stretch the tissues around it and restore or increase movement. Often an area of the body becomes contracted after an injury and mobilisation can be used to restore the normal movement by stretching the ligaments and muscles that hold the joint in place.

Manipulation

Manipulation is similar to mobilisation but stretching of the joint is applied more quickly. This enables the muscles around the joint to remain relaxed allowing the joint ligaments rather than the muscles to be stretched. Manipulation can be used to release tightness in joints caused by shortening of the joint ligaments. During the technique you may hear a pop. This is due to the joint unlocking as tight ligaments are stretched, allowing the joint to move more freely.

Traction

Traction is another technique that seeks to stretch the joints open, and is most commonly used to treat people with a trapped nerve causing pain down an arm or leg. Stretching open the joint helps to release pressure on the nerve.

Acupuncture

Acupuncture has been shown to be effective in treating muscle and joint problems and is frequently used as part of a programme of treatment. Acupuncture encourages healing by stimulating blood flow and the release of positive chemical factors.

Exercise Regimes

Chiropractors, physiotherapists and osteopaths may advise specific exercises to assist recovery from back or neck pain. When people find themselves incapacitated due to their injury or following an operation, exercises can restore fitness by building muscle stamina and strength. Where an area has become very stiff, stretching exercises may be advised to loosen it. For a joint which has become inflamed and irritable, exercises involving repetitive, gentle movements can be used to ease the problem without aggravating it.

Posture, work and lifestyle

Where a problem is chronic a chiropractor, physiotherapist or osteopath can provide insight and advice on how posture, work and lifestyle factors may be affecting your condition, and offer suggestions for improvement.

Manual therapies – safe and non-invasive

In the treatment of back and neck pain, medical guidelines recommend the use of manual therapies as described above, because they are safe and non invasive.

Which is the best technique?

No single, physical therapy technique can be regarded as superior to another as each patient responds differently, moreover some types of injury are easier to treat than others. For instance, a condition that is easy to treat may respond equally to several different approaches, while a more difficult injury may require a specific combination of techniques. Confronted with a difficult injury an experienced practitioner has the expertise to tailor treatment to ensure the best outcome.

Your Family Doctor

Initially most people consult their family doctor when they have a health problem. However if you have back or neck pain, the most common cause is some form of joint strain. The healthcare professional most qualified to treat back and neck strains are chiropractors, physiotherapists and osteopaths who have specific training in this type of injury.

Symptoms which may indicate a condition other than a back or neck injury

We need to be mindful however, of other types of harmful conditions which can give symptoms of back or neck pain such as infections, cancers and kidney disorders. Although these types of condition can present symptoms of back or neck pain they are much less common than a simple joint strain.

Indicators that pain is due to something other than a joint strain

You can look for indications that you may have something other than pain due to a simple joint strain. These are, feeling unwell, loss of appetite, changes in bowl or bladder activity, having a temperature, finding your pulse is more rapid than normal, or other physical changes that are unusual. In such cases it is advisable to consult your family doctor.

Mild back pain – medical advice

Once your family doctor has confirmed that you do not have any of the above symptoms, it will become apparent that your problem is some form of common back or neck injury. If you are not too disabled by pain and able to function more or less normally your doctor usually advises that the pain is likely to subside eventually and until then to cope as best as you can. This is perfectly sensible advice, a high proportion of mild back and neck strains will resolve without any treatment. An even higher percentage will settle if managed correctly,

The do's and don'ts for back and neck strains

I have outlined management of back and neck strains and the do's and don'ts in Chapter 1 (back pain) and Chapter 9 (neck pain).

Treatments for back and neck pain available from your family doctor

In this section I will explain the different kinds of treatments that are available from your doctor for the relief of neck and back pain. In the case of significant pain your doctor may prescribe any of the following individually or in combination: anti-inflammatories, pain killers and muscle relaxants.

Anti-inflammatory

Most types of tissue injuries that cause back or neck pain involve some degree of inflammation therefore, anti-inflammatories such as ibuprofen, naproxen, or diclofenac sodium, may help to relieve the symptoms and are recommended in national guidelines on treating back pain.

Pain killers

Anti-inflammatories do not suit everybody, for instance people with asthma or hypertension may find their problem exacerbated. Anti-inflammatories can also cause stomach irritation and other side effects. In these cases pain killers are often prescribed.

Some people find taking painkillers helpful because painkillers enable them to move about and attempt gentle activities such as walking, which they could not attempt otherwise. In other sections of this book I have recommended gentle movement of the back joints as a means of easing the symptoms of back pain. In cases of severe pain where the individual is unable to find any position that is comfortable and feel tired and tense through lack of sleep, painkillers can be helpful.

Risks of long-term use of painkillers

It is not advisable to rely on painkillers in the long term. If your condition fails to improve, I recommend seeking further assistance rather than continue to take painkillers. With prolonged use pain killers can become addictive and can cause serious side effects. Some patients have reported constipation or nausea after using codeine based painkillers for only a few days. If you are able to find a comfortable position to rest in and can stand up and move around, however slowly without too much discomfort, then painkillers will probably not improve your situation significantly. If you can manage without them you are not at risk from harmful side effects.

Muscle Relaxants

Muscle relaxants are often prescribed for back or neck pain. Recent studies however, suggest muscle relaxants may not be as helpful as previously thought and in some cases may delay recovery in patients with low back pain. Muscle relaxants such as diazepam work by causing sedation. Sedation reduces the individual's level of activity and this lowering of activity levels is thought to be the cause of muscle relaxants giving poor results in some studies of their use in low back pain. However if your pain is very severe and you find muscle relaxants taken at night help you sleep, then their sedative effect may be of some benefit.

Orthopaedic/Spinal Surgeon

Many people suffering from back and neck pain consider the orthopaedic/spinal surgeon to be foremost in treating back and neck problems. Although in a small number of cases intervention from an orthopaedic/spinal surgeon will be beneficial, studies show that surgery is appropriate in less than 0.5% of cases of back pain. Consequently, the majority of family doctors presented with cases of common back or neck pain tend to advise against an initial consultation with an Orthopaedic/Spinal surgeon because professionals such as chiropractors, physiotherapists and osteopaths are more likely to be able to offer assistance.

Treatments for back and neck pain available from the orthopaedic/spinal surgeon

The cortisone injection

A common treatment for back or neck pain by the medical specialist is the cortisone injection. When a joint has been irritable and inflamed for a long period, the inflammation can become self-sustaining, which means the body finds it difficult to settle the inflammation on its own. In many cases anti-inflammatory tablets are ineffective. This could be because medication absorbed from tablets relies on the blood stream to carry them into the injury. Some tissues in the body such as ligaments and tendons have a poor blood supply which limits the amount of drug that is delivered through the blood.

A common solution is to inject the anti-inflammatory directly into, or close to, the affected tissue. This method ensures a high dose in the area where it is needed. Normally a steroid anti-inflammatory is used mixed with a small amount of local anaesthetic for greater effect. Various injection approaches may be used to place the drug directly around the inflamed part of the joint.

The main types of spinal injection

Sacral epidural injection

In this type of injection an opening at the bottom of the sacrum is used to introduce the drugs into the spine. This method is often used when the patient has both low back and leg pain.

Nerve root injection

In this case the injection is inserted into an opening at the side of the spine where the spinal nerves come out. This method is also used for people with back and leg pain.

Facet joint injection

The facet joints are parts of the spinal joint that lie nearer the surface of the body than the discs. Pain from the facet joints is usually accompanied by tenderness over their location, about 1 inch (2.5cm) to the side from the centre line of the spine.

Sacroiliac joint injection

This injection is usually done into the lower part of the sacroiliac joint. Pain felt in the sacroiliac joint can often be referred pain from an injury to the low back. In difficult cases a sacroiliac injection can be useful to differentiate between a low back problem and a sacroiliac problem.

General use of cortisone injections

Cortisone injections are also used in many other areas of the body for chronic inflammatory pain, such as the shoulder and elbow. It is normally considered a straightforward and safe procedure. While there is no guarantee that it will work for every patient it can be of help in some cases. Steroid injections are also used to help with diagnosis. If the injection reduces the pain, then the area of injury is confirmed and if necessary can also be targeted with other treatments.

Surgical treatments for back and neck pain used by the Orthopaedic/Spinal surgeon

Discectomy

Other treatments used by the orthopaedic/spinal surgeon for back pain are mainly surgical. The most common of these is the discectomy which is used when some material from a distorted disc is pressing on a nerve. The position of the problem is located with an MRI scan and then a small incision is made in order to remove or clean out the material that is pressing on the nerve. If an accurate diagnosis has been performed then this can be a very successful operation.

However even though you may have a damaged disc which has been confirmed by an MRI scan, using a surgical procedure to treat it is not normally the first option. This is because, firstly the majority of disc problems will resolve with other forms of treatment, and secondly because surgery has a higher risk of complications compared to other forms of treatment. For these reasons most surgical specialists will often suggest an initial course of manual treatment such as Chiropractic, Physiotherapy or Osteopathy.

Surgery is recommended only when all the other sensible options have been explored, or if the disc is causing highly debilitating pain or interfering with other body functions.

Laminectomy

A laminectomy is another surgical technique used in patients with nerve compression. A laminectomy is used when nerve compression is caused by bony protrusions forming around the facet joints at the rear of the spine rather than from a disc, a condition known as spinal stenosis. In this procedure part of the back of the spine and any extra bony nodules are removed to relieve pressure on the nerve.
A laminectomy is also sometimes used with a very badly damaged disc as it allows better surgical access to perform a discectomy.

The symptoms of spinal stenosis can be slightly different from a slipped disc. Although both often produce back or leg pain, or both. In spinal stenosis the symptoms are usually at their worst when standing and walking whereas with a slipped disc the symptoms are normally worse when sitting.

Posterior lateral inter-body fusion (PLIF)

Other more technically demanding surgical procedures may be used to treat spinal conditions, such as the posterior lateral inter-body fusion (PLIF). This can be used with a discectomy or laminectomy and incorporates metal plates secured across the back of the spine connecting the bones each side of the damaged joint. Because these plates take the stress off the joint and stabilise it while the joint is healing, the patient is able to become fully mobile more quickly.

The orthopaedic/spinal surgeon – the initial consultation

What to expect

The initial consultation with an orthopaedic/spinal surgeon is usually brief and consists of an assessment to determine firstly, whether any treatment they offer is appropriate and secondly, if it is necessary to arrange further investigation such as an MRI scan.

Describe your problem clearly and accurately

Be aware that the surgeon's assessment of how serious your condition is will be based on what you describe. Avoid a brave front and playing down your difficulties which can mislead the surgeon into thinking your problem is less severe than it actually is. For instance, saying, "The injury is quite painful but I am managing to work." creates the impression of a low degree of pain. Whereas, "Although I am still working because I am self employed but I am in pain all day and afterwards my back is so painful I hardly get any sleep." informs the surgeon your pain is severe. Describe your symptoms accurately, and in particular which movements aggravate your symptoms and which normal activities they prevent you from doing. In short how your quality of life is affected.

Find out what treatment is offered

Ensure you are informed about the treatment the orthopaedic/spinal surgeon can offer. The surgeon may suggest surgery or some kind of injection. The prospect of having a surgical procedure or injection may be a cause of anxiety. Prior to seeing a surgeon I recommend preparing yourself by finding out what treatment the surgeon may offer. If you have been referred by a healthcare professional they can tell you what you need to know before your appointment. Being informed will help you to feel prepared and able to consider all your options.

Case Study

A patient came to my surgery with a problem that I diagnosed as being caused by severe wear of one of his hip joints. Because the wear in the hip was so advanced I would normally advise consulting an orthopaedic surgeon with a view to having the hip replaced. The patient however, had already seen a surgeon and declined the offer of surgery. We discussed the procedures available to him. Following the discussion he admitted that had he been better informed about the choices open to him he would have felt more confident about choosing a surgical procedure.

Patients have the right to refuse treatment, but in my experience many patients decline treatment because they are inadequately informed about the treatment options they are offered.

Chapter 12
Additional exercises and information

Exercises for Flexibility and Good Posture

Exercise is vital to improving posture and helping prevent low back pain.

Many people bend from the waist, but the spinal joints in the waist area are not designed to absorb the stress of bending in this way so they can be easily strained.

Exercises which help prevent bending from the waist are particularly effective in preventing low back pain because they reduce the stress on the spine caused by bending incorrectly.

Please note
People who are suffering from acute back or neck pain should refer to appropriate sections earlier in the book.

Bending correctly prevents low back pain

When bending, muscles around the waist area should come into action and contract. This serves two purposes firstly, to support the back and secondly, it stiffens the waist to prevent bending occurring at that point. When reaching over to pick something up, bending should occur mainly at the hip joints. The hips are the strongest joints in the body and the ones most capable of coping with bending stresses. If the hip joints are tight and lack full movement it will be difficult to bend correctly at these joints, which can cause people to start to bend from the waist instead. Injuries of the spine most frequently result though straining the spinal joints at the waist level.

Maintaining correct natural bending movements

Patients frequently seek advice on exercises to prevent low back pain. I cannot emphasis enough the importance of establishing good reactions in the core muscles around the pelvis and flexibility in the hip joints. Both these are essential in assisting correct natural bending movements that protect the low back area from being overstressed.

Good posture depends on maintaining flexible hip joints

Bearing this in mind the following general flexibility exercises focus on the hip joint. Not only is flexibility in the hip joint essential in order to bend and lift correctly as mentioned above, but also because the hip joints are the largest joints in the body, and the largest muscle groups are attached to them. As a result any tightness in the hip joints will manifest in all the major muscle groups and through them affect the whole posture.

To a large extent keeping the hip joints relaxed and mobile keeps the whole posture relaxed.

An abbreviated exercise programme - good for those with little free time

Throughout I have emphasised the benefits of good posture and how it may be achieved. Firstly, through keeping the hips flexible and relaxed to ensure the low back and pelvis are not tense and secondly, by keeping the rib cage, mid and upper back, loose and lengthened so the upper body is not slumped forward.

The amount of time devoted to maintaining flexibility depends on your natural flexibility, as well as your age.

When time is limited, I recommend concentrating on some of the exercises with legs supported by a wall for the hips and some stretching exercises for the mid and upper back. All these exercises are described later in this chapter.

Skin Brushing or Patting – good for warming up

These exercises gently warm up the muscles, loosen the joints and stimulate the nervous system. They involve brushing or patting the body with the palm of the hand.

When brushing aim for a feeling similar to rubbing your hands together to create static electricity. Try to use one continuous movement, relax and try to avoid rushing.

When patting aim for a soft feeling with the hand and arm relaxed moving slowly over the body. Spend a few moments working each area.

Below I have included two routines which together cover the whole body. If time is limited you can use the technique of brushing or patting to loosen and stimulate any area of the body.

Exercise

Brushing and Patting Arms - good for loosening shoulders and upper back.

To start straighten the arms out in front with palms facing each other and held loosely together.

From this position move one palm up the front of the other arm into the shoulder. If your shoulders are relaxed as you move your palm up the inside of the arm, your arm will naturally swing backwards and rotate slightly outwards.

Now move the palm over the shoulder and down the outside of the arm to the back of the hand, over the finger tips so the palms meet again. As you move the palm down the outside of the arm, if you are relaxed you will find the arm swings forward and rotates slightly inward again.

Repeat the cycle for a few minutes without stopping.

Additional exercises and information

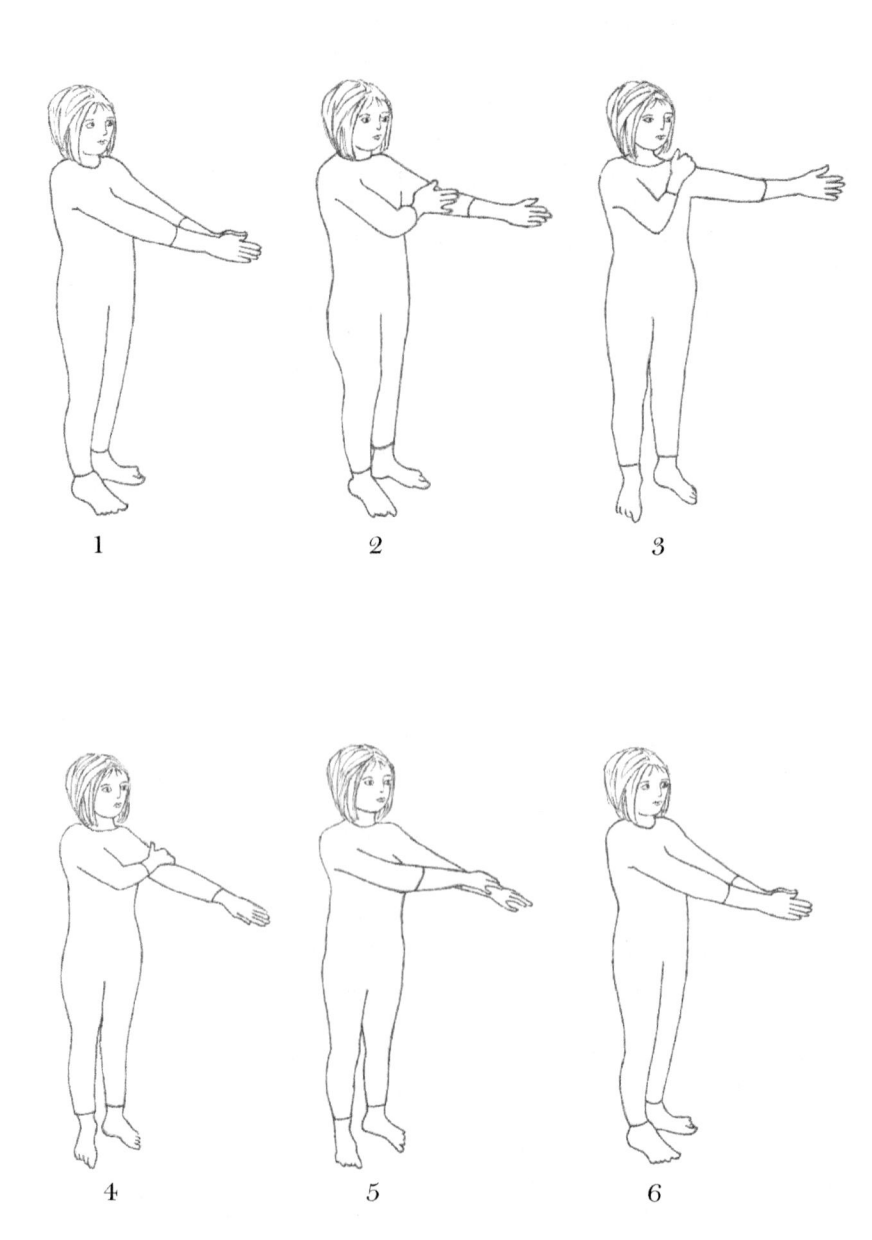

1 2 3

4 5 6

Additional exercises and information

Brushing the body and legs - good for loosening the hip joints, improving strength and stamina in the low back, buttock and pelvic muscles and encouraging a natural bending technique

This exercise is done in one continuous movement.

To start place the palms on top of the head moving them down the back of the head to the back of the neck.

Without pausing move the palms around the sides of the neck to the front of the body. Continue brushing your palms down the front of the body, keeping palms each side of the centre line until you reach the waist.

From the front of the waist move each hand simultaneously around the side of the waist to the small of the back into the kidney area.

Now bend carefully at the hips and bending the knees keep the back straight with the head in line. From the low back area move the palms over the buttocks and down the back of the legs as far as you can without straining while keeping your back straight.

Most of the bending should occur at the hips, the knees should not bend further forward than the front of the feet.

At the furthest point down the back of the legs you can reach, comfortably move the hands round to the front of the legs and continue brushing back up the front of the legs, body and face to the top of the head again.

Do repetitions of the exercise cycle for a few minutes.

Although this exercise is primarily for the lower back it is essential to include the upper body part of the movement. This not only stimulates and loosens the upper body but more importantly, brushing up the body and over the top of the head ensures you straighten up fully. The action of straightening up fully before bending forward again is highly beneficial for the low back joints.

Additional exercises and information

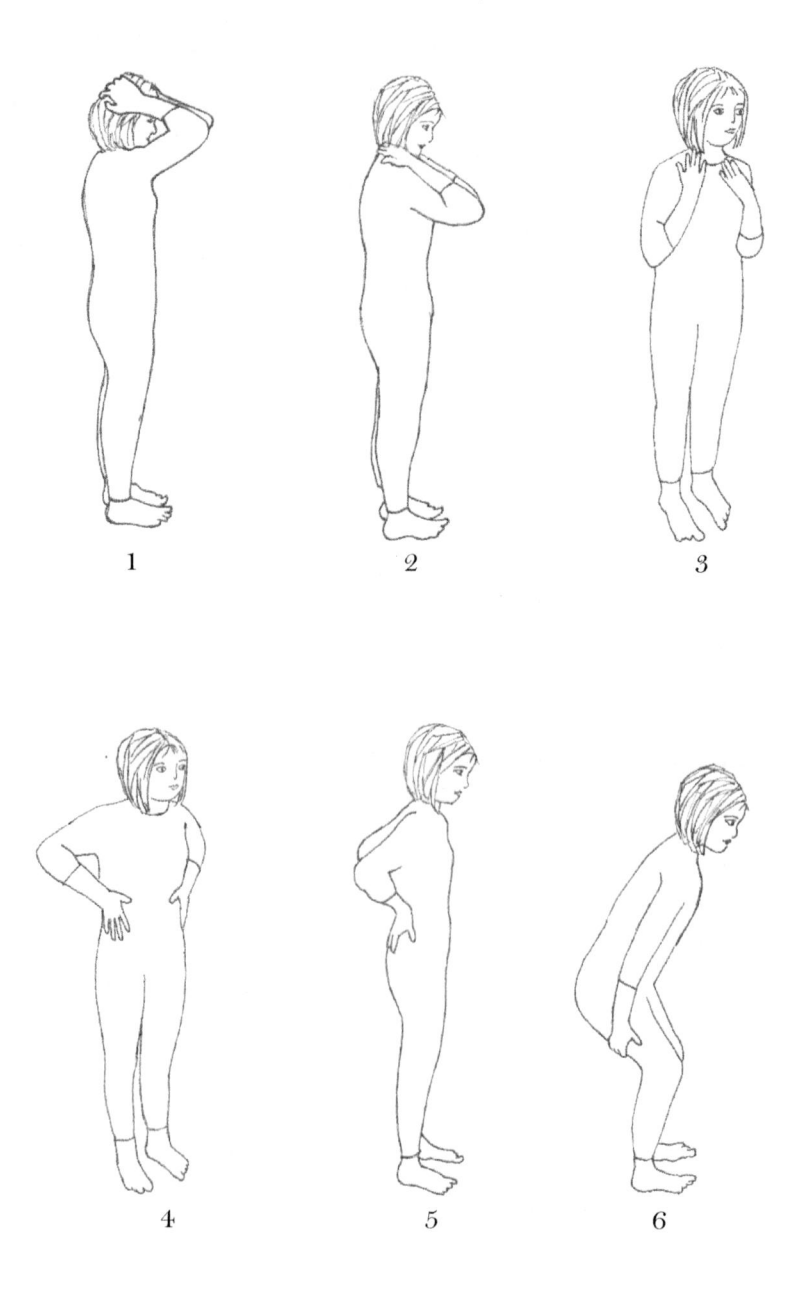

1

2

3

4

5

6

162

Additional exercises and information

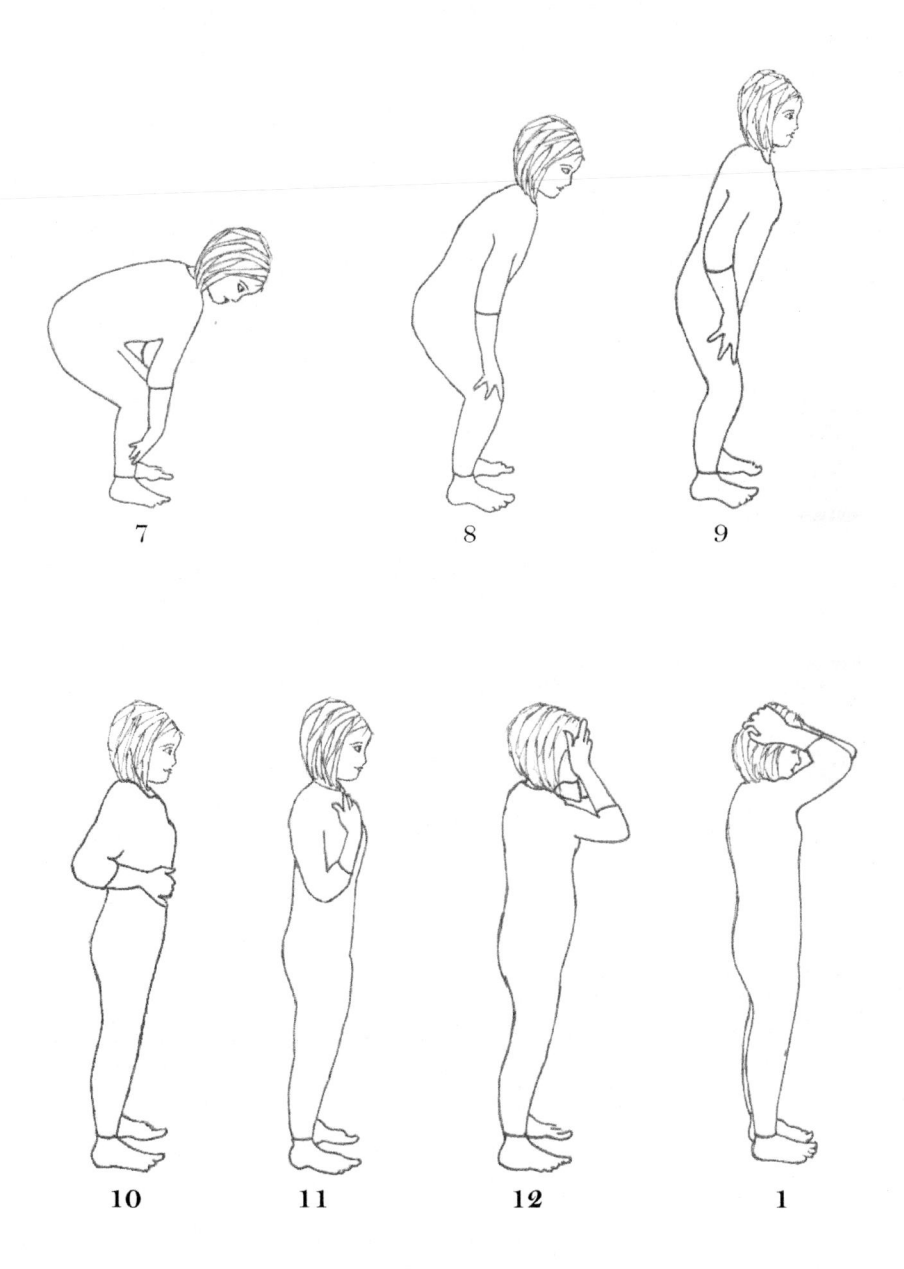

7 8 9

10 11 12 1

163

Exercise

Both legs raised against a wall or door (four simple exercises)
Good for loosening low back, pelvis and hips
Good for people who run or play a sport regularly

Exercise 1

This exercise is particularly beneficial, stretching the back of the legs, pelvis and hips and involves very little effort. It also places very little strain on the low back, and is therefore better for people with a history of back pain, compared with stretching the legs by bending forward from the standing or sitting positions.

To start lay on your back with your hips placed close to a wall or door with legs raised against the wall or door, knees bent slightly. I recommend a painted door to avoid marking the wall.

Slowly straighten the knees and pull the toes toward you to produce a stretch.

Move the hips toward the wall for a stronger stretch.

Avoid being too close to the wall and attempting too strong a stretch, which will cause your legs to feel uncomfortable and can result in pins and needles if you attempt to hold the stretch for any length of time.

Rest in this position for four or five minutes, or as long as it remains comfortable.

Doing this exercise regularly helps loosen the low back, pelvis and hips.

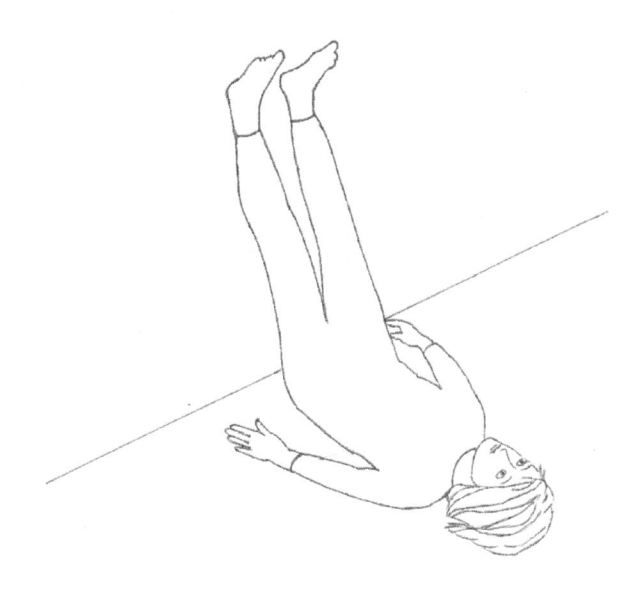

Modified exercise – raising one leg at a time
Good for people with low back pain.

The exercise above can be modified for those with a sensitive low back by raising only one leg at a time.

To start raise one leg against the door frame of an open doorway while placing the other leg along the ground through the doorway.

Continue the stretching action as in the previous exercise using one leg at a time.

The modified exercise produces less rotation and strain in the pelvis and lower back, and can be useful if those areas are very sensitive.

Modified exercise – placing legs slightly away from the wall
Good for improving core muscle response and stamina

To start raise both legs against the wall, bring one foot a few inches away from the wall and hold for 5-10 seconds.

Now do the same with the other leg.

Repeat up to ten times each side.

This exercise strengthens the pelvic muscle groups.

If you can hold this position comfortably, hold both legs slightly away from the wall to work the muscles more strongly.

Additional exercises and information

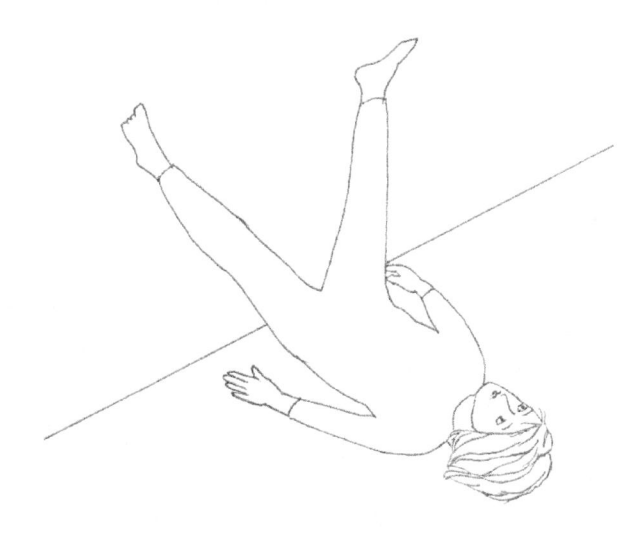

Exercise 2 - good for stretching the inner leg muscles

To start raise both legs against the wall, allow your legs to open and slide apart.

Unless your hip joints are very stiff there should come a point where the weight of each leg starts to pull it down.

At that point you can relax and let gravity do the work stretching the hips and muscles on the inside of the legs.

Stay in this position for four or five minutes or as long as it remains comfortable.

Exercise 3 – good for stretching hips and pelvis

To start raise both legs against the wall, allow your knees to bend and your feet slide down the wall as far as is comfortable.

Let the knees fall apart, then relax your legs letting their weight stretch your knees further apart until you feel a stretch in the hips and pelvis.

Stay in this position for four or five minutes or as long as it remains comfortable.

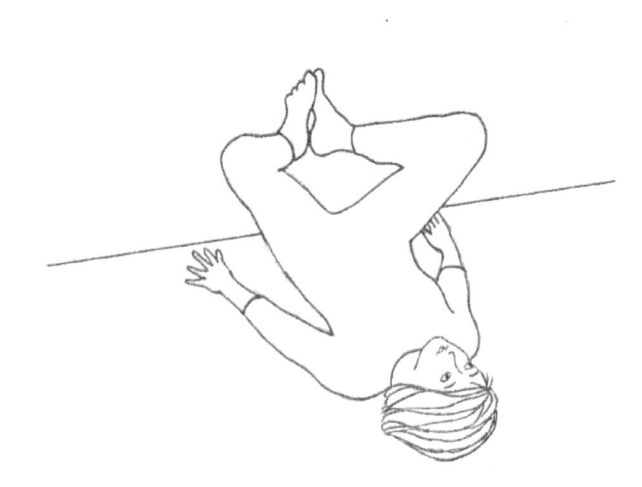

Please note if wall exercises cause discomfort

Staying in these stretches against a wall for as long as four or five minutes can be uncomfortable for some people. To alleviate any discomfort hold each exercise for less time and alternate between the exercises several times.

For instance, doing one of the above exercises for one or two minutes then changing to another of the exercises for one or two minutes and then swapping back again.

Repeat this cycle until you have accumulated 4 or 5 minutes in each exercise.

If there isn't enough time to do all these exercises for 4 or 5 minutes or you find them uncomfortable try starting with 2 or 3 exercises. Alternatively stay in each one for a shorter time.

Exercise

Specific hip stretches – good for tightness in the hip joints

Particularly beneficial for:
People who run regularly or play sport
People with osteoarthritis and restricted movement in the hip joints

The hip stretches are good for people with restricted movement in their hip joints. For example people who run regularly or play a sport which involves a lot of running such as football, often have tightening of the hip joints. Similarly, in older people tightening of the hip joints is common due to osteoarthritis of the hip joints.

Please note if you have had a hip replacement
These exercises may not be suitable for people who have had a hip replacement. Please seek individual advice as repetitive stretching of artificial hips can destabilise these joints.

Additional exercises and information

Exercise

Specific hip stretch 1 - good for tightness in the hip joints

To start lie on your side on a comfortable surface. Place a pillow under your head to protect the neck from strain.

Bend the lower leg as this helps keep the position stable. Lift the top leg straight up, keeping it in line with the body.

When you have gone as far as you can comfortably, give a little extra stretch upward for one or two seconds then lower.

In this exercise there are two points to consider, firstly as you lift the leg up there is a tenancy to bring it forward and not keep it in line with the body. Doing this will raise the leg further but you will loose some of the stretch in the hip.

Secondly, make sure you relax the leg completely in between each repetition or you will cause the hip joint to tense up.

Do approximately ten repetitions once or twice a day.

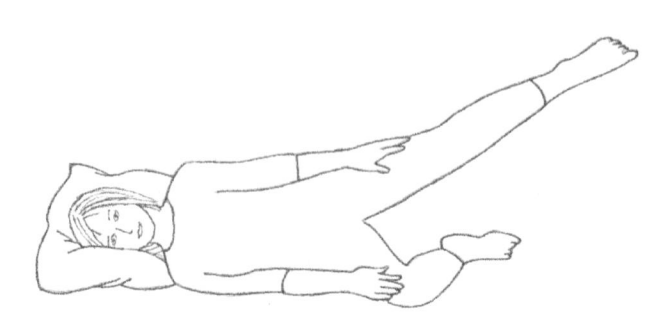

Exercise

Specific hip stretch 2 - good for tightness in the hip joints

To start lie on your side on a comfortable surface. Place a pillow under your head to protect the neck from strain.

Bend your top leg forward from the hip keeping the leg and the knee locked straight. When you have gone as far as you can let the leg rest down on the floor for a few seconds still keeping it straight.

If it feels awkward to drop the foot to the floor place a cushion to support the foot so the leg does not have to drop too far.

After a few moments resting with the leg forward, bring the leg back and keeping the leg as straight as possible swing it behind you. Rest it on the ground when you have gone as far as you can comfortably. Again a pillow can be placed on the ground to support the foot if it feels uncomfortable.

After a few moments resting in this position bring the leg forward again and repeat the stretch.

Do approximately ten repetitions once or twice a day.

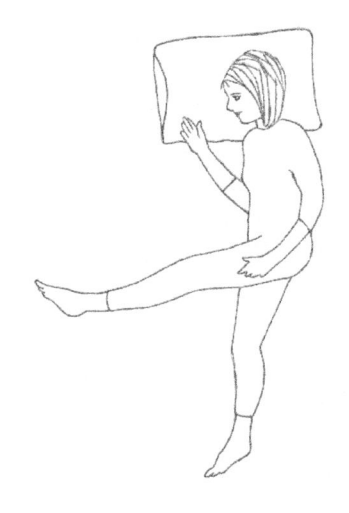

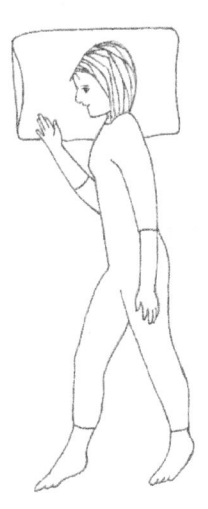

Additional exercises and information

Exercise

Stretching backwards – good for stretching the front of the legs, knees and ankles

For this exercise you need to be fairly flexible in your hips and knees therefore it may not suit everyone.

To start kneel down and sit on your feet with knees together in front of you. Make sure the inside of the feet lie next to each other and the bottom of the feet face upward.

This position provides a good stretch for the front of the legs, knees and ankles.

If however this position causes discomfort, place a cushion on top of your feet to raise yourself up and reduce the stretch on the front of the legs and knees.

If you can sit on your feet comfortably in this position you can increase the stretch on the front of the legs by leaning backwards against a chair or cushion.

If you are very flexible you can lean backwards until you are resting on the floor. To protect your back please take care to use your arms to lower yourself backwards onto the floor.

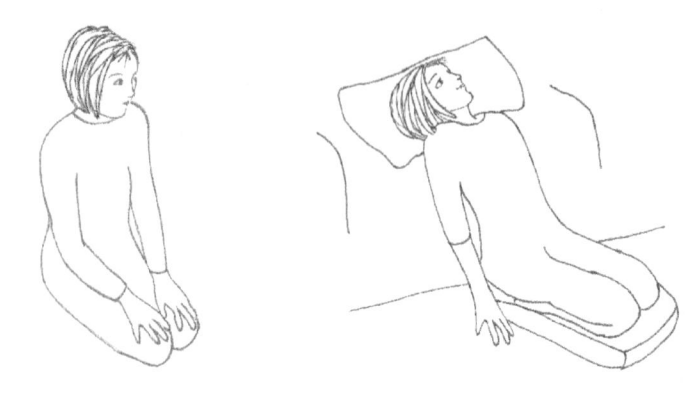

Exercise

Crossed leg stretch – good for hip Joints

To start sit on the ground or on a cushion cross legged. If you are not very flexible, sitting raised on a cushion makes this exercise easier.

With your legs crossed relax your knees down as far as possible. Cross your arms and then with each hand hold the opposite knee.

Using your arms pull yourself gently forward over your legs.

Hold for about 3 breathes.

Now cross your legs and arms with the opposite leg and arm on top and repeat.

Repeat two or three times in each of the two positions.

The exercise provides a stretch in the hip joints and across the top of the back.

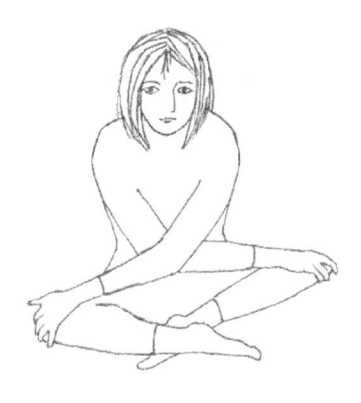

Additional exercises and information

Exercise

Side stretch – good for loosening the rib cage, upper back and shoulders

To start adopt a standing position, place 90% of your weight on one leg. Keep enough weight on the other leg so you can remain balanced easily.

On the side where you have placed most of your weight lift the arm over your head and stretch to the opposite side, at the same time keeping 90% of the weight on that leg.

Hold the stretch for 3 or 4 breaths. It can be repeated 3 or 4 times to each side.

Keeping most of the weight on one leg while stretching to the opposite side, stiffens the waist area. This causes the stretch to be felt more in the mid back and side of the rib cage.

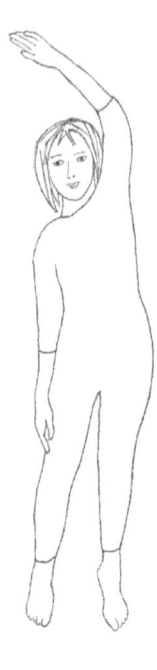

Stretching and loosening the rib cage is highly beneficial as in most people it tends to be tight. A tight rib cage causes the whole of the mid back, upper back and shoulders to be restricted.

The exercise on the previous page can be done from a starting position with the hand palm down or palm up. Each hand position gives a slightly different stretch down the side of the body.

Exercise

Strong upper body side stretch – good for those with a good level of flexibility

Providing you have a good level of flexibility, you can increase the stretch in the side of the body by doing the previous exercise while seated.

Depending on the level of flexibility in your hip joints, you can do the exercise from a chair, sitting raised on a cushion, or sitting on the floor. The higher your seating position the easier it is.

To start place one leg outwards to the side you are going to stretch towards, as far round to the side as you can. Keep it straight and ensure the other leg is relaxed with the knee bent.

Now gently twist your body a little away from the outstretched leg so that the outstretched leg is in line with the side of the body. Lift the opposite arm over your head and lean toward the outstretched leg. You should feel a good stretch down the side of your body.
Hold the stretch for 3 or 4 breaths. It can be repeated 3 or 4 times to each side.

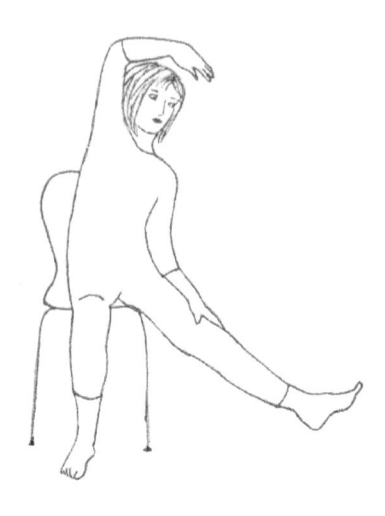

Sit-ups

Can I do sit-ups when I have back pain?

Sit-ups are a popular exercise and patients often ask if it is advisable to do sit-ups while suffering from back pain. I would advise caution in doing sit-ups with back pain as they can be jarring to the low back. If you have a history of back pain I would recommend the following precautions.

Do sit-ups slowly

Sit-ups can jar the back if done too quickly. Taking your time with each sit-up is more important than trying to achieve a high number quickly. Doing fewer repetitions but at a slower pace can be just as effective.

It is much easier to lower yourself down from a sit-up slowly than raise yourself up into it slowly. Therefore it is better to take more time lowering yourself down out of the sit-up than raising yourself up into it.

Avoid raising yourself too far

Avoid coming up too far, lifting your shoulder blades off the floor is far enough, lifting further tends to make your back muscles tense up and has little added impact on the stomach muscles.

Keep your head in line with your back

Try and keep your head in line with your back and avoid bending the head forward.

Placing your hands behind your head to support it during sit-ups will help keep your head in line with your back and reduce neck strain.

Additional exercises and information

Keep your low back relaxed during sit-ups

If you have a sensitive back it is especially important to keep your low back relaxed while doing the sit-ups. Not coming up too far, not flexing your head forward and not doing the sit-ups too fast will help.

Keep one leg straight and the other with knee bent up

Another useful strategy to help keep your low back relaxed while doing sit-ups, is to keep one leg straight on the floor and the other with the knee bent up. You will find this helps stop flattening and tensing of the low back while doing sit-ups.

Strenuous exercise, warming up and winding down

Warming up – good for increasing muscle reaction

Warm up exercise should warm up the body because warm muscles can absorb oxygen from the blood stream more easily and can react faster metabolically to produce energy quicker.

Static stretching, that is holding areas of the body in a stretch, fails to warm up muscles adequately. The best method of warming up is either jogging or brisk walking for 5-10 minutes, or some kind of dynamic exercise that warms and loosens the areas that are going to be used most in the activity. For instance, arm circling or leg swinging.

Winding down - good for avoiding dizziness

During exercise the heart rate increases and blood vessels expand to promote blood supply to the muscles being used. Stopping suddenly may result in dizziness. This can be avoided by winding down during the last 10 minutes and doing the exercise at a slower pace. Alternatively you can exercise at a slower pace, by jogging or walking.

Stretch after winding down

Following the last 10 minute winding down period is the best time to stretch. At this stage your muscles are still warm which is an ideal time to stretch to improve flexibility. On a cold day it may be best to do stretches in an indoor space so that the muscles remain warm.

Feeling sore after strenuous exercise is normal

Soreness after exercise is caused by slight damage to muscle fibres produced during use. A warm up or cool down routine cannot prevent this, therefore it is normal to feel sore after strenuous exercise.

Using heat or cold to encourage healing

In answer to the frequently asked question "Should I use heat or cold on my injury?" the two main factors to consider are, the depth of the injury and how inflamed it is.

Deep injuries

Heat or cold applied at the surface will not penetrate far into the body. Therefore, if you have a deep injury such as a slipped disc or deep ligament strain, applying heat or cold at the surface will have little direct effect on the injury. However, because applying heat or cold can be comforting it is worth doing, the pleasant feeling it produces distracts from the pain which helps the area relax.

In a deep injury it doesn't matter whether you use heat or cold, use whatever feels most comfortable.

Treating an inflamed injury

In an injury where the damaged tissues are near to the surface of the body and the area is very sensitive to touch or pressure, the choice of hot or cold depends on the amount of inflammation.

Inflammation is an irritant because it involves the release of chemicals in the area of the damaged tissue. Heating these chemicals up makes their irritant nature more pronounced which is why the advice often given is to cool an inflamed injury.

Reducing the temperature suppresses chemical activity within the inflammation, reducing the irritation it produces.

Applying an ice pack

Cover the inflamed area with a thin piece of material about the thickness of a thin T shirt or blouse to prevent the cold irritating the skin. Then apply the ice pack for 5 to 10 minutes once per hour. Normally an injury will be acutely inflamed for the first forty-eight hours which is when using a cold pack is most effective.

However because cold reduces biological activity and blood flow, using a cold pack after the first forty-eight hours may slow down the healing process. If an injury still feels inflamed after forty-eight hours, another option is to use contrast bathing.

Contrast bathing

Contrast bathing consists of using hot and cold packs alternately, for about 5 minutes each. This causes the blood vessels in the area to expand and contract, stimulating blood flow in the injury without allowing too much heat to build up. You can rotate between hot and cold 2 to 4 times.

When contrast bathing start with the hot compress such as a hot water bottle, and finish with the cold ice pack to remove heat at the end.

A few final words

The information and practical advice compiled in this book are based on my experience with patients who suffer from back and neck pain. Drawing on the information and advice I provide my patients on a daily basis I have compiled an accessible, self help guide to pain relief.

The guide is intended for use at home, to remind patients of the recommended advice and exercises which they can follow to assist their recovery.

I have avoided unnecessary jargon, making the information and advice concise and easy to read.

Posture and exercise - the key to a healthier life

In compiling this guide to pain relief I wanted to draw special attention to the importance of posture and exercise in maintaining health. Knowing about exercise and posture and how to use our bodies efficiently leads to a more efficient use of our energy and effort in our daily activities. Efficient use of our bodies enables us to do more, feel less tired and prevents possible injury.

Exercises - an easy to follow programme

The recommendations and exercises contained in the book demand very little time, making them ideal for people with busy lives. You can easily select one of the simple exercises to practice for just a few minutes and with very little effort increase your wellbeing.

Following more of the advice and exercises will increase your understanding of how to use your body more efficiently. Using your body efficiently will increase energy and enable you to improve your participation in everyday activities, and ultimately enjoy a fuller life.

Printed in Great Britain
by Amazon